THE DENTOFACIAL COMPLEX

Lectures of Dr. Allan G. Brodie

Edited by
William S. Bike, Dr. Arthur H. Craven,
Dr. Lawrence Furstman,
and Dr. Raymond C. Thurow

United States Copyright Office
Certificate of Registration
TXu968-823

Published by UIC College of Dentistry Press,
Office of Advancement, 801 S. Paulina, M/C 621,
Chicago, IL 60612-7211, (312) 996-8495.

ISBN: 0-9710459-3-3

Printed in the United States of America

CONTENTS

Foreword:
Dr. Allan G. Brodie

The best student Dr. Edward Angle, the "father of orthodontics," ever had, Dr. Allan G. Brodie (1897-1976) came to the University of Illinois at Chicago College of Dentistry in 1929 to start the graduate program in orthodontics.

His seminars quickly became renowned for the quality of his teaching; his writings were avidly read; and his example attracted scores to teaching and research. His own theoretical research set his reputation as a scholar as firmly as his use of the edgewise arch established his clinical renown.

Adding administrative excellence to that reputation, Dr. Brodie served from 1929 to 1966 as orthodontics department chair and from 1944 to 1956 as the College's dean and orthodontics chair simultaneously.

Internationally known as a clinician, teacher, administrator, and researcher, Dr. Allan G. Brodie set the standard for orthodontic expertise through much of the 20th century.

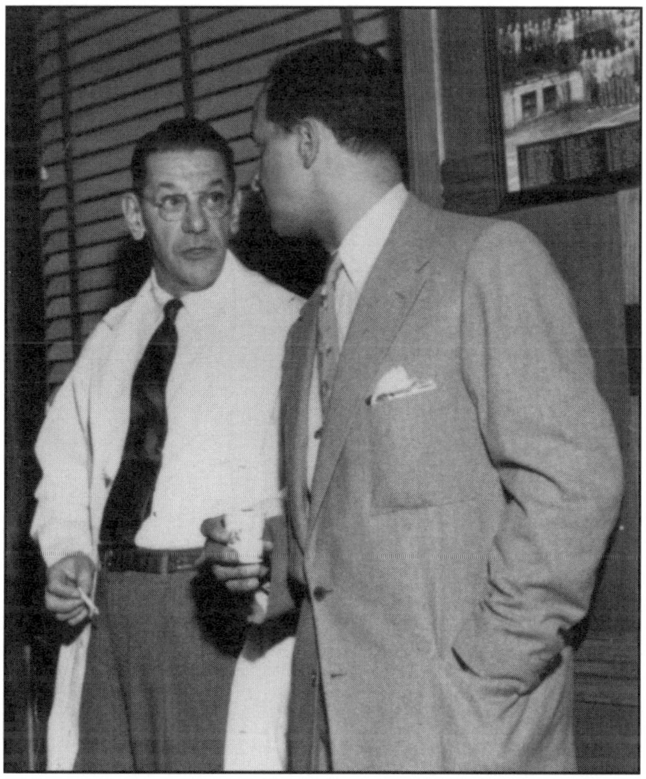

Fig. Foreword-a. Dr. Allan G. Brodie Sr. (left), discussing Department of Orthodontics business with longtime fellow faculty member Dr. Earl W. Renfroe (right).

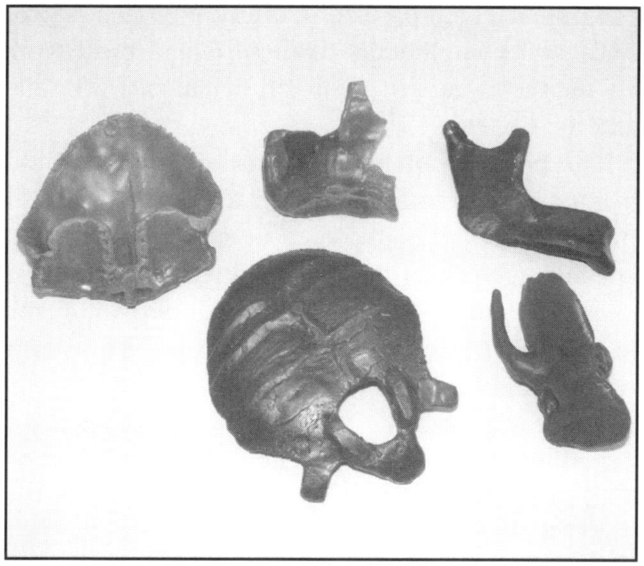

Fig. Foreword-b. Dr. Brodie assigned exercises to orthodontic specialty students in which they carved model craniofacial bones from red wax.

"Dr. Brodie had the ability to elicit a positive, energetic, and forceful response from his students," recalled one of them, Dr. Bernard J. Schneider, who earned his DDS degree from the UIC College of Dentistry in 1954 and his MS in orthodontics from the College in 1956, and who is a faculty member at the College.

"He taught by example and he taught by scholarly activity and wide frame of knowledge," Dr. Schnieder continued. "I can remember sitting spellbound in one of his early seminars and whispering to one of my classmates, 'This man wants us to think!'"

Late in life, Dr. Brodie began work on putting a series of his lectures together in book form. After his death, several of his former students and colleagues continued the effort, which became this book.

Arthur H. Craven, MS ortho '52, DDS '54; Lawrence Furstman, DDS, PhD, ortho '34; Raymond C. Thurow, DDS '44, ortho '47, did yeoman work in writing, editing, and choosing illustrations before the book, *The Dentofacial Complex,* came to my hands. In addition, Andrew J. Haas, DDS, MS ortho '58, was the driving force in organizing the process and in keeping the project going during difficult times. Drs. Carla Evans, T.M. Graber, Gerald Borden, Cyril Sadowsky, J. Daniel Subtelny, Benjamin H. Williams, and Abd El-Moneim Zaki, and Ms. Margaret Bjerklie, also assisted. On behalf of the UIC College of Dentistry, I am pleased to offer the College's gratitude and compliments to these dental professionals for their years of effort on behalf of Dr. Brodie and the College.

The book is compiled as Dr. Brodie would have written it, with information left intact that has later been supplanted or replaced by new knowledge. It is a time capsule of the orthodontic knowledge that existed through Dr. Brodie's career, providing the benefit of a rich historical background to today's orthodontic teaching.

To provide benefit to students, the public, and the profession, the UIC College of Dentistry has created the Allan G. Brodie Institute for Orthodontics. The Brodie Institute extends the College's Department of Orthodontics' excellence beyond teaching to research, patient care, and service to the profession, "a think tank that will be a combination Mayo Clinic and National Institutes of Health of orthodontics," according to Dr. Carla Evans, head of orthodontics at UIC.

The Institute emphasizes scholarship and research, resulting in even higher-quality teaching as breakthroughs are immediately added to the curriculum.

That emphasis beyond teaching attracts both the finest students and the finest faculty. The Brodie Institute increases the value of a UIC orthodontics education for alumni as well, not only through enhanced reputation but through the Institute being a center of excellence for pathbreaking continuing education.

We think Dr. Allan G. Brodie would be proud of both this book and the Institute, both of which are honored to bear his name, and are created to make one think—just as Dr. Brodie would have wanted.

William S. Bike
Associate Director for
Advancement and Alumni Affairs
University of Illinois at Chicago
College of Dentistry

Preface: The Dentofacial Complex

The dentofacial complex is at once the most vital and one of the most intricate parts of the human body. It presents the portals for food and air and the end organs for sight, hearing, and olfaction. Each of these has been brought to its present level of perfection by adaptations of its own and between it and other structures.

It should not be surprising that an area with such varied functions would be the object of attention of an equally varied assortment of health professionals; each of these must of necessity limit the scope of his or her efforts in order to insure the attainment of a high level of competence.

The limits of a field are usually established on the basis of treatment procedures, e.g., surgery, orthodontics, or on the basis of a clearly delimited area such as the nose and throat. But such limits on the area of operation cannot be placed on the knowledge of the specialist. Therapy applied to even the smallest area should be based on the understanding of the etiology of the problem and the overall consequences of the therapy. In an area as complex as the face the interrelationships are broad and numerous.

'Diagnosis is a matter of more than measurements and tables, or simple observation. It must encompass a total understading of the patient's problem in relation to age, heredity, and environment.'

Diagnosis is a matter of more than measurements and tables, or simple observation. It must encompass a total understanding of the patient's problem in relation to age, heredity, and environment. The immediate problem must be considered in relation to its causes and the ensuing consequences that have succeeded it as well those that can be expected in the future. Therapy, as a means of altering these circumstances, must be considered in the same light.

This book is an effort to provide a broad view of the dentofacial complex. What it is, what it does, where it came from, and the ills to which it is heir are all matters for our interest and concern. Perusing the titles of the seminars, the casual reader would be apt to think that, because he or she has studied much of the material before, it can be applied immediately to his or her specialty. The reader quickly finds he or she has not retained the knowledge in sufficient completeness to serve in this manner without a careful review of old and the addition of new material.

The author's own search for understanding of the biological processes which underlie orthodontic problems brought him in contact with all of the other dental specialties, many in medicine, and such related fields as growth, anthropology, histology, and speech. Throughout his entire teaching career at the undergraduate, postgraduate, and graduate levels he has included material derived from such sources in his lectures and seminars in an effort to cultivate in the dental graduate an appreciation of such a background. This cannot be accomplished by lectures alone. It requires a method that insures serious participation of student discussions. Seminars meet this requirement better than any other method of

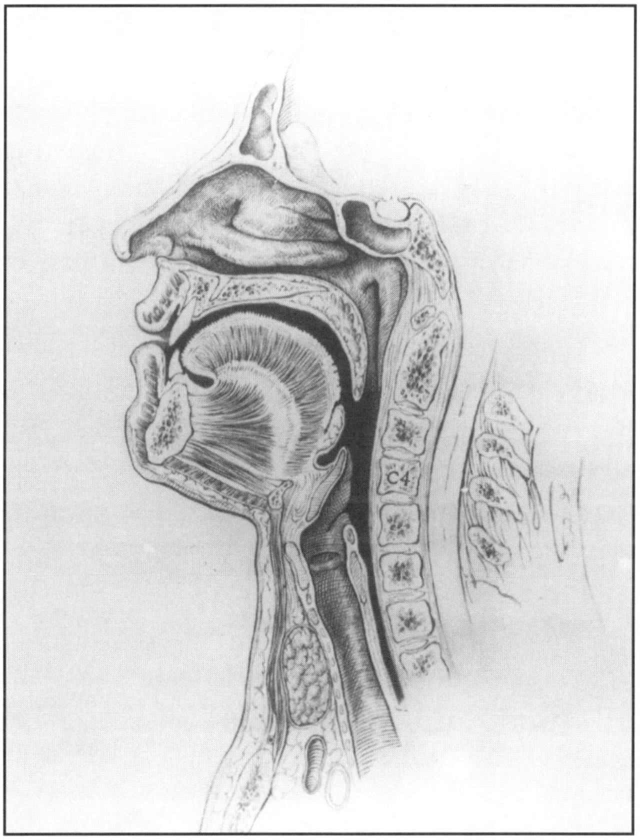

Fig. Preface-a. Section of head.

pedagogy.

Obviously it would be impossible to cover in a book a seminar course in orthodontics as it actually transpires. The reports, the comments and discussions, the questions and answers, chalk sketches, and the flashes of humor are matters of but a fleeting moment and have meaning only for those who participated. Any effort to preserve the course as a unit is doomed to failure, as was shown by recording a number of them. But the students who took part in them for nearly 40 years have been well-nigh unanimous in the opinion that the seminar was their greatest learning experience. It is upon their urging that I have attempted to salvage what I could from texts, reprints, theses, notes, and memory and put them into a semblance of order that might be understandable and helpful to a reader, whether teacher or student.

Unfortunately, it is not possible to convey by the written word several conditions that contribute significantly to the effectiveness of the seminar method. Like all clinical fields, orthodontics lacks a foundation of its own. It rests entirely on a base of biologic sciences. The means to ensure that a reader possesses a knowledge of the facts and principles of those sciences are not available to a writer, whereas assignments, quizzes, and tests can be used by the teacher. Further than this, probing serves not only to refresh the students' memory of subjects he or she has studied in the past but also, if handled in combined quiz-seminar fashion, to indicate the difference between memorizing material and utilizing it to develop concepts. These advantages are denied a reader and their lack saddles a writer with the dual responsibility of handling both recall and integration. To overcome these deficiencies to a partial degree, reading lists have been strategically placed throughout the book to enable the reader to find the sources of the material covered.

Thus we see that the prime purpose of the seminar method, the Socratic approach, is to encourage the student to think rather than assimilate facts uncritically. As has been said so wisely, "Any man who has been taught to any purpose has been largely his own teacher."

Allan Gibson Brodie

1. General Biological Principles

It is well known that all life resides in protoplasm, which can be broken down into its inorganic constituents: carbon, nitrogen, oxygen, etc. As biologists, we also appreciate that such a chemical analysis does nothing to explain the special manner in which these elements combine to impart those characteristics called "life" which set protoplasm apart from the non-living world. Organic and physical chemistry indicate that protoplasm is organized in the form of relatively large protein molecules which are constantly reacting with those around them in many different ways and at speeds that were not comprehended only a few years ago. This intense activity never results in a static equilibrium, but rather in a continuously responsive dynamic equilibrium (homeostasis), which operates within definite limits.

The organized unit of protoplasm is the cell, usually thought of as a circumscribed mass surrounded by a membrane. This membrane is not to be considered a skin, but only as a chemical modification of the cytoplasm itself, resulting from its contact with the extracellular environment. Indeed, if a part of the cell is sliced off, the cut surface immediately assumes the role of a semipermeable membrane.

If viruses are excluded, cells are the smallest living units with specific needs for food and oxygen for survival. Further, cells must be able to react to select what is good for them, to avoid that which is harmful, to assimilate foods into their own substance and, since this activity inevitably results in end products, they must be able to excrete wastes. To maintain the continuity of life, they must reproduce. All of these activities constitute the so-called vegetative phases of existence; they are organized to support the life of the cell without reference to other cells. They are directly related to the cell's interdependency with its environment.

It now becomes useful to think in terms of a membrane containing the cytoplasm of the cell. Everything upon which the cell depends must come from without itself. Food, oxygen, and stimuli flow into it from the environment and wastes flow out into the environment. The avenue of entrance and exit is the cell surface. The cell is thus vitally dependent on the area of its surface for all its needs.

A new cell is small and can grow. But this growth means an increase in three dimensions with volume increasing by the cube, while the surface of the cell increases in only two dimensions or by the square. If the cell membrane is thought of as working at top capacity to supply the contents of the cell, it will be apparent that a limiting ratio must exist between a unit of surface area and the unit of volume which it can support. In the new cell, the ratio is high in terms of surface and low in terms of volume but, as size increases, this ratio decreases steadily in terms of the surface related to increasing volume. Eventually a point is reached at which surface area balances metabolic demand. To grow further is impossible, because it would mean the death of the cell. The cell can obtain more surface area only by dividing. Such division seems to take place with the attainment of certain sizes in different cells, small cells usually being characterized by high activity and frequent division.

Multicellular Organisms

When cells divide they tend to remain together, although there are exceptions such as the amoeba. The size of aggregates of cells which would result from the division of individual members soon meets the same limiting factors as those faced by the individual cell, since only cells at the periphery are in a favorable location for supplying their needs from the environment. By what adaptations was this handicap overcome so that the multicellular organisms could survive to grow and progress?

A number of living forms yield clues to the various methods that evolved in answer to the need. The simplest of these consisted of corrugations, invaginations, and evaginations of the surface of the cell mass which permitted the environment to reach deeper into the interior. Another was the adaptation of tube-like forms, the walls of which consisted of only two layers of cells. Still another witnessed the development of openings penetrating in all directions throughout the cell mass. Such forms were extremely weak structurally and came to be supported by a spicular framework such as we see in the sponge. In all of these there was a tendency toward cell specialization to the end that those cells in direct contact with the environment became adapted for more efficient absorption of nutriment.

This progression to higher multicellular forms witnessed the development of an internal circulating system which has established communication between the environment (surface of the tube) and cells lying remote from it. This metabolic system became the carrier of food and oxygen and the conveyor of wastes, effectively removing the basic limits upon the size and form to which an organism could evolve.

The Postulates of Organic Evolution

Before going further, it seems wise to pause and examine the manner in which these basic functional modifications are thought to have come about. The process is evolution, propounded by Charles Darwin, which rests on four main postulates:

I. *Multiplication.* Simple forms of animal life give rise to enormous numbers of offspring. These might be looked upon as so many experimental situations.

II. *Variation.* No offspring are identical to any other or to the parents. Some are better, while some are more poorly endowed to cope with the environment in which they find themselves.

III. *Competition (survival of the fittest).* Fitness in this sense means ability to support life in the environment in which the organism finds itself. It must compete with such factors as temperature, atmospheric pressure, gravity, sunshine, etc. in addition to other forms like itself. Thus, the environment determines which will survive.

IV. *Irreversibility.* Any given organism gives rise to more fit and less fit progeny; one might assume from this that a less fit form might give rise to one that was more fit and in this way regain lost ground. This does not occur. Any new trait, once it has appeared, tends to breed itself into a stronger form; hence an undesirable characteristic tends to become even more unfavorable to the point that it may become lethal. Obviously the favorable characteristic tends to strengthen itself, making the animal more fit, so long as the environment remains stable.

Selective Breeding of Plants and Animals

When organic evolutionary matters are under consideration, there is a tendency to think teleologically, viewing changes as responses to a need rather than occurring by chance alone. Any change in organic form represents only one of many that occur, but it is the one that happens to prove successful in meeting a need that is most likely to capture our attention.

Advantage is taken of Darwin's postulates, particularly number IV, in the breeding of plants; corn offers an excellent example. The breeder has in mind certain characteristics he wishes to strengthen such as drought resistance, disease resistance, size, number of rows of kernels, sweetness, and late or early maturity, when he makes his first planting. Having sown his seeds, he leaves them without irrigation, cultivation, or care of any kind. Regardless of the occurrence of unfavorable environmental conditions during the growing period (drought, disease, flooding), some of the plants will probably survive. With such indications of resistance to whatever unfavorable conditions have operated, the next planting is made from the seeds of the survivors. These plants are even more resistant to the undesirable conditions which operated on the first planting. In addition, there may have been new factors on the second sowing which have affected it. A third planting is made from survivors of previous plantings and so on, progressively breeding desirable characteristics into the seeds.

The same postulates govern man's efforts in animal breeding. Here the wish may be to increase the yield and/or quality of meat and milk in cattle, the speed of race horses, the size of turkey breasts, and the reinforcement of the myriad characteristics of dogs. The breeding of animals for such purposes, however, is accompanied by certain risks. Too persistent inbreeding for a trait by the mating of two animals superiorly endowed with a given feature frequently results in offspring which are lacking in other valuable or even essential characteristics.

The same strengthening effects which are sought for the desired characteristics will operate with equal effectiveness on unwanted qualities which may also be present.

Adaptations Leading Toward the Vertebrates

The increasing complexity of animal forms does nothing to reduce demands of the environment; indeed, the reverse is true. Hence, the appearance of mutations which led to the ability to move were bound to have advantages since such a power would endow its possessors with the possibility of seeking new environments.

Changes in Body Form

Cell masses in a water environment tend to assume a spherical form which is a definite handicap for motion. Adaptation toward elongation was one step in the direction of oriented movement but this change in shape, to be advantageous for self-induced movement, required changes in other systems and tissues. The supporting framework which had already appeared in such forms as the sponge now showed definite reorganization by a longitudinal arrangement in the middle of the body. This body exhibited bilateral symmetry in those forms whose accompanying adaptations would make self-induced movement possible.

Specialization of Tissues

Since the specialization of tissues had progressed a long way in certain systems such as the food- and oxygen-procuring cells, it was necessary that other functions be taken over by special groups if the animal were to be successful in obtaining food instead of depending on water currents to bring it. The special sense organs that would eventually lead to the detection of food by sight, olfaction, hearing, and feeling, together with the great center to receive and sort the stimuli coming from these end organs, all began as more sensitive areas of the outer covering. Ultimately they gathered at the forward end of the animal, which is the first part to enter a new environment. With them was associated the orifice that was to procure the food and the oxygen to burn it. And with all these there was the development of a system that was capable of causing self-induced movement: the muscular system. This constituted the basic vertebrate pattern which was to be the ground plan for all later forms.

The Vertebrate Pattern

The early vertebrate had already attained polarity; it had taken on an elongated form and was destined to continue this change until it also became "streamlined" with the greater part of its bulk at the forward end and tapering toward the tail or caudal end. This tear-drop form is the least resistant to movement through water or air and provides a fulcrum for the tail. Simultaneously, it derives the greatest aid for movement from the environment, thus conserving energy.

Running the length of the body was the vertebral axis, a flexible rod of tissues derived from the parental mesenchyme, and to this were attached the first muscles of movement. Being disposed symmetrically, these muscles balanced each other and by their alternate contraction acted to bring about undulations of the body. At this stage this was apparently their sole function and the main function of the vertebral rod itself. Since the animal lived in water, its environment provided his support. Thus, little added strength was required of its skeletal muscles.

At the center of the forward end of the column were gathered the primitive brain and the end organs of the special senses. The eyes were situated at the side of the head covering a visual field of 180 degrees above the animal which at this time was flat dorsoventrally and lay on the floor of the sea. The olfactory area of the brain was located between the eyes on the top of the head where the environment reached it through an opening in the surface.

The otic area, destined eventually to become the organ of hearing, lay behind the eyes and consisted of a membrane capable of detecting differences in the pressure of the surrounding water.

All of these end organs together with the brain that was to receive their stimuli and translate them into patterns of activity were supported and separated from each other by supporting, modified connective tissue. These supporting "baskets" together with the vertebral column constituted the endoskeleton.

Along with the adaptive changes noted above were modifications that were to give the animal protection. These are thought to have arisen through the development of an increasing toughness of the outer skin that culminated in shagreen. Shagreen covered the entire body and head and, in some forms, developed into plates of various sizes that constituted an armor similar to that which characterized the crustaceans.

In the line of animals that was to progress to higher forms, this plate-like covering persisted only in the head region, leaving the body unemcumbered and therefore allowing for greater quickness in movement. It should be realized that, with the development of an outer covering, the animal was now the possessor of both an endo- and exo-skeleton. Both features were destined to undergo further modifications and to remain contributors to the crania of all higher animals.

From all the foregoing, certain fundamental conclusions can be drawn.

I. It is the environment that is the main if not the sole determinant for the survival of living forms.
II. Slight variations in every characteristic of offspring result in either increased or decreased "fitness" or compatibility with the existing environment. Such variations in the organism are due to chance alone.
III. Both favorable and unfavorable variations are strengthened in subsequent generations. The first contributes to advancement, the second to extinction.
IV. Development of the special senses furnishes living forms with the means of detecting food and enemies. Each of these senses evolved independently according to the nature of the environment and the availability of food.
V. Food is but a part of the essential demands for organic life, oxygen being equally important to convert the food into energy. It is the pursuit of energy that is the chief concern of all life and the efficient utilization of that energy is as critical as its procurement.

Every possible device for the conserving of energy can be found associated with each adaptive change. Such devices range from the equilibrium between muscle forces and gravity to the metabolic activity of cells. The oceans have constituted a far more stable environment than have the land masses. The latter cover a relatively small area of the Earth's crust, which is essentially a shell covering a molten core. That vast movements have taken place between the crust and the core and between the crust and the sun is indicated by the profound differences that exist today between the polar and equatorial regions. Present conditions may be complete reversals of those of earlier ages. Equally great have been the changes between and within the land masses that have witnessed the rise and fall of the continental shelves, the thrusting up of mountain ranges, and the development of the polar ice caps.

Each of these cataclysms has resulted in the elimination of all but the more generalized forms of terrestial life of the time. Thus, those animals that became adapted to their environment were unfit under the conditions imposed by new environments.

Reading list:

Darwin, Charles. *The Origin of Species.* New York: Grammercy, 1998.

Darwin, Charles. *The Descent of Man.* Princeton, N.J.: Princeton University Press, 1981.

Gerard, R.W. *Unresting Cells.* New York: Harpers Brothers, 1949.

Jones, Steve. *Darwin's Ghost.* New York: Ballantine, 2000.

Thompson, D'Arcy. *On Growth and Form.* Cambridge (England): University Press, 1952.

Weiss, Paul. *Principles of Development.* New York: Henry Holt & Co., 1939.

2.

The Evolution of the Mouth Parts and the Lungs

Until this point little has been said about the structure that has long been characteristic of the cephalic end of the emerging vertebrate animal. This is the orifice leading to the gut, the stomadeum. It attained definitive characteristics probably with the development of the exoskeleton. The respiratory system underwent changes associated with these developments.

The exoskeletal plates came to cover not only the outer surface of the head, but also the lining of the anterior part of the gut, so that a bony orifice or mouth was formed. In back of this cavity there were wide apertures on either side leading to the gill arches, cartilaginous bows festooned with highly vascularized membranes. The water taken through the mouth was pumped over these capillary beds by action of the jaws so that its oxygen could be absorbed.

The plates covering the head and jaws of this early animal were numerous and simple in form. To provide the general overall sheathing there were special groups associated with different functional parts. One group of plates surrounded the eyes, another the otic area, and two roofed the snout and ran from the margins of the jaws to the brain covering. These were quite large in the early facial complex, although they were destined to be reduced to relative unimportance as they later became the nasal and lacrimal bones. The evolutionary history of the entire exoskeletal head is one of reduction of the number of component bones with an increase of complexity of the surviving members. This is strikingly demonstrated in the complex architecture of the bones of the human head. Each is involved in a number of functions and these functions are reflected in the form, structure, and relationship to other bones of the facial complex which are responsible for vital functions, i.e. nutrition, respiration, and communication.

For the purposes of the present review we chiefly are interested in those bones that came to be concerned with the teeth, the dentaries which developed into the mandible below and the maxillary complex above. All were originally insignificant, channel-like bones that covered the margins of the stomadeum. The dentaries (right and left) below were supported by sixteen pairs of plates and in the maxilla and premaxilla by the numerous bones of the upper face. It was on the margins of these original sheathing bones adjacent to the orifice that teeth first appeared, but it should be pointed out that at this stage there were two jaws, the lower contained within the upper.

The lower jaws resulted from a forward bending of the most anterior gill bars which were associated with the pumping of water over the gills. Being already provided with musculature for this function, they were readily adaptable to the opening and closing of the stomadeum. The development of the sheathing bones with spines that were to become teeth provided the animal with a great advantage in grasping the slippery prey on which he lived. Indeed, this advantage proved so great that it is speculated to have been the chief determinant in the development of the face which Gregory called "a glorified fish trap."

Beginning as small elevations of the shagreen, the teeth, proving valuable, evolved rapidly. The centers of the small shagreen elevations first hardened and then began to be elevated forming higher and sharper spines. It is possible that, eventually, such high spines were too delicate and too poorly attached to withstand the increasing strain put upon them. Thus, further adaptations probably contributed additional modifications of their attachment to the jaws, beginning originally with direct ankylosis. Perpetual succession of teeth in some species emerged as another factor of insurance, so that, if a tooth was torn off, another formed in its place.

The strengthening of the jaws came about through the increasing dominance of the inferior dentary (mandible) and the maxilla and premaxilla. These three bones continued to increase in size and strength, developing in a superior and posterior direction displacing the smaller supporting bones until contact was made with the sheathing bones of the brain case. Contact between the mandible and the brain case, with the development of a temporomandibular joint, was not accomplished until the age of mammals (Fig. 2a).

The Emergence of Living Forms in an Air Environment

It is intriguing to speculate upon the conditions that resulted in living forms leaving their watery environment and adapting to survival in the Earth's atmosphere. Such speculation must take into account the new conditions that they faced and the adaptations that were necessary for survival and further evolution. Among the demands that had to be met were (1.) the ability to absorb oxygen from air, and (2.) the ability to adjust from a physically partially supportive environment to the forces of gravity and to atmospheric pressure.

In water, a living form derives great assistance from its environment for support and movement in space. With a body density similar to the surrounding water, such living creatures were maintained in position with little expenditure of energy. In movement, most energy could be devoted to the contraction of controlling muscles supported by the environment and aided by its body design. In the Earth's atmosphere, on the other hand, the animal was subjected to the forces of gravity and received no aid from the environment, carrying the increased load produced by gravity and atmospheric pressure. Thus, these two forces were added to the environmental factors with which the eventual land animals had to adapt.

Some of these forces tended to flatten the early forms of living organisms against the Earth's surface. Had they been capable of generating enough energy to erect themselves, they would still have been unable to do so because of the weakness of their skeletal framework. Thus, two further important developmental adaptations were essential, viz. (1.) the mechanism for obtaining greater amounts of nutrition and oxygen to supply the increased energy demand, and (2.) the strengthening of the skeletal system. This second demand required less dramatic changes and was met by a calcification of a cartilaginous skeleton that was already formed, but the first demand required widespread physical modifications. The obtaining of greater amounts of nutrition and of oxygen necessary to metabolize it required modification and increased efficiency of the alimentary and respiratory systems which were devoted to these functions.

The respiratory system will be considered first in interest of continuity, with the alimentary system discussed later when the tooth apparatus is studied. It is not definitely known how the internal lung began, but there is strong evidence that some vertebral forms had progressed a long way toward air breathing before they left the water. Some of the transitional stages between the water and air breathing creatures are generally thought to be various forms of lung fish still living in Australia, Africa, and South America.

The African form Protoperus has been the subject of the most study and seems to offer the most logical evidence of this transitional stage. It has an air bladder that develops embryologically from the gullet much as the lungs of higher vertebrates do. In the early fish it was supplied with air by the gills and it served as a hydrostatic organ to accommodate the animal to the pressures of different depths of water. In Protoperus this air bladder is a paired structure running the full length of the body cavity with a lining that is highly vascularized. Thus, in water it continues to act as the hydrostatic organ, while in air it can act as a lung. In water with insufficient oxygen, it can supplement its oxygen as the goldfish does by gulping air at the surface of the water. Indeed, this particular lung fish can survive for long periods of inactivity out of water. When the shallow water in which it lives evaporates in the dry season, it buries itself in the bottom muck, curls up, and breathes through a small aperture; thus it stays alive from one wet season to the next.

It is believed that the air-breathing lung of terrestial animals evolved through the branching of this air sac within the thoracic cage, ventral to the gut. This provided more and more surface for the abstraction of oxygen from the air that was brought to it. Again, the necessity of surface to the environment proved the important condition to progress. The demands for oxygen were not limited, however, to those made by support and locomotion; indeed, these were relatively small because they really constitute only a small part of the need for oxygen. The biggest demand is for heat production.

The metabolism of animals living in water is adjusted to the temperature of the water. Some fluctuations of water temperature are slight due to its high specific heat, the metabolic rate is kept at a fairly constant level, and all bodily functions are carried out most efficiently at that temperature.

Animals on land which are dependent on the

environment for the level of their metabolic activities have only to return to the water if the temperature of the air drops. Failing to do this they suffer a sharp drop in their metabolism and become inactive. Such is the case of the amphibians which are capable of airbreathing but are not able to rely completely on their oxygen intake for heat production.

Those animal forms which were to survive and remain active in air had to adapt in such ways that they could obtain vastly increased amounts of oxygen and food for the increased energy demanded by a heat regulating system. The mere intake of greater amounts of nourishment and oxygen would do no good unless it were directed to maintaining a level of body temperature sufficient to make the animal independent of the temperature of its environment. A simple example from elementary chemistry will serve as an illustration.

If you dissolve sugar in water at room temperature you ultimately reach a point at which no further sugar can be dissolved. However, if you now raise the temperature of the water you find that more sugar will be accepted. Ultimately, a temperature is reached beyond which no more sugar can be added; a point of maximal solution has been reached.

So it is with the dissolving of oxygen in hemoglobin. There is a point of temperature at which a maximum interchange takes place and, as might be surmised, this temperature is close to 98°F degrees in humans. Anything that disturbs this level by as little as two or three degrees throws the entire body metabolism out of balance and affects all systems. One could imagine what would happen to an animal with a drop of 20 degrees if he were not buffered against it. Small wonder that the adaptations of animals to air breathing is looked upon as one of the greatest advances in organic evolution. And, small wonder that the adaptations it demanded were so extensive. They involve not only the tremendous increase in surface area of the lungs but equally profound changes in the skeleton of the face, as will be seen later.

In the first chapter certain phases of the phylogeny of the head were considered and it was pointed out that the beginnings of movement on the part of early, water-living forms was one of the chief determinants of the vertebral form of organization. This form was elongate and symmetrical and gave direction to movement. It was likewise of extreme value for survival that the end organs of most of the special senses should be gathered at the forward end since it would be upon these that the animal would depend to locate food and avoid enemies. The special senses are the first parts to enter a new environment.

As each of these organs evolved, it was supported and protected by specialized tissues around it so that the group that ultimately formed the head in the beginning could be looked upon as a relatively loose collection of parts that were individually well advanced. Each was connected with the central nervous system. The food and oxygen procuring mechanisms can be thought of as lying separately from the special sense organs. Both were served by

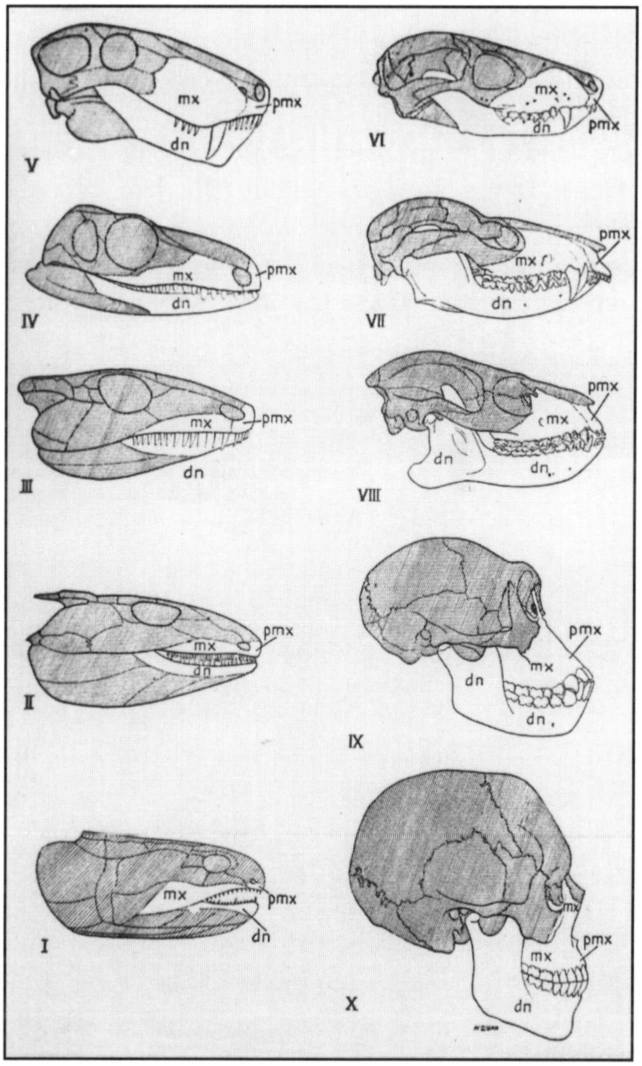

Fig. 2a. Reduction of bones of the face and jaw as the many small bones of the jaw became reduced to form the mammalian mandible and maxilla.

a special group of bones which constituted jaws and which helped to form a stomadeum. The stomadeum acted as a portal or trap for both food and oxygen.

Since energy enters the body as food and oxygen, the parts responsible for the gathering and utilization of these essentials had to be enormously increased in efficiency. Although teeth had already appeared, they were poorly attached. Now, they became complex in design and were supported by bone to withstand the stresses put upon them. A loosely organized head skeleton would no longer serve as a foundation against which they could function, and this was likewise strengthened.

The gill arches could not supply sufficient oxygen to serve the increased intake of food, and the respiratory system adapted accordingly. A slit had appeared in the ventral wall of the gut, and this led to a closed pouch capable of holding a small quantity of air. This pouch began to spread down inside the thoracic cage and to lobulate until it offered vast surfaces for the absorption of oxygen.

The Devonian lobe-finned fish had already evolved holes in the bones covering the anterior part of the jaws between the premaxillae and lacrimal elements. These led into a space above the palate. Part of the water, mixed with the food gulped by the animal, passed through these nasal pits. Entering this bypass off the mainstream to the gut it was slowed, permitting scents to be detected by the olfactory centers of the brain which were situated, then as now, just above the scent-bearing stream. From here the water rejoined the mainstream to the gut through an aperture in back of the palate which at this time was continuous with the dorsal wall of the gut, thus providing an opening between what was to be the nose and the gut.

This served olfaction admirably since the streams flowing through the nasal pits passed over the olfactory lobes of the brain. At the same time it would bring about a crossing of the food and air tracts at a lower level. This necessitated a valve to prevent both being open simultaneously when the animal became completely dependent on air for oxygen. The valve which evolved was the larynx.

Reading list:

Gregory, W.K. *Man's Place Among the Anthropoids.* Oxford, UK: Oxford University Press, 1934.

Gregory, W.K. *Evolution Emerging.* New York: Macmillan Co., 1951.

3.
Functional Evolution of the Larynx

We refer to the region behind the oral cavity as the pharynx and should recall that, since the vertebral column is essentially horizontal, the roof of the pharynx is the dorsal wall of the gut. It was in this wall that an anterior aperture developed to provide communication with what came to be the nasal chamber above the palate.

Previously were described the early adaptations that occurred in the ventral wall or floor of the gut to form a slit that developed into an aperture leading into a pouch, which was divided into two sacs. The branching and elongation of these sacs provided an enormous increase in vascularized surface for contact with the oxygen-bearing medium within the thoracic cage.

This chapter deals with the crossover of the alimentary and respiratory tracts in the pharynx and the mechanism to avoid the entrance of any substance other than air into the respiratory system.

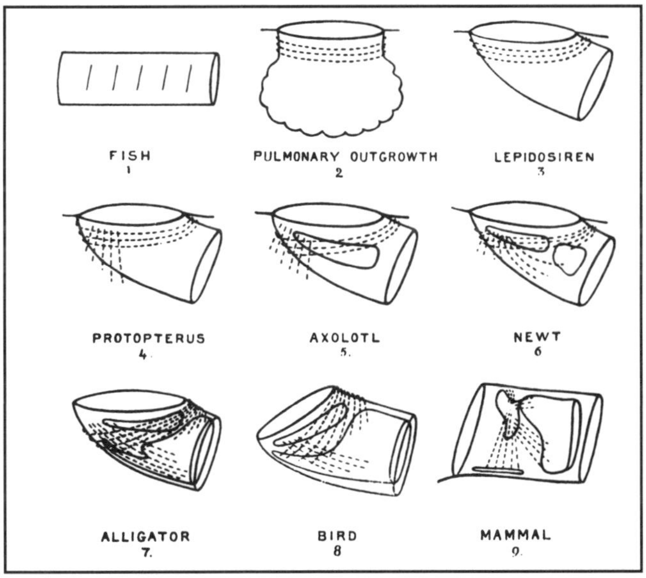

Fig. 3a. Stages of development of the pharynx.

According to Negus, the aperture between the sacs and the pharynx was adapted through a series of stages illustrated in Fig. 3a. In the first four stages the opening was controlled only by closure through simple sphincter action, but with stage 4 there was the beginning of positive, muscular dilation. Stronger and more positive control over dilation was given in stage 6 with the appearance of the arytenoid cartilages in the wall of the sphincter. Later stages witnessed further strengthening through the appearance of the thyroid and cricoid cartilages.

The epiglottis did not appear until the age of the mammals, but it was destined to become of vital importance to all higher animals. Its role was that of providing a valve between the air and food channels so that both could not be open at the same time. During inspiration, the air stream had to be directed from the aperture in the dorsal wall of the gut to that in the ventral wall, crossing the pharyngeal part of the gut.

In early forms the integrity of the air stream is assured by an elevation of the bronchial tube through a sphincter in the soft palate where it is held whenever the mouth is closed. It is retracted and closed when the jaws are closed and when

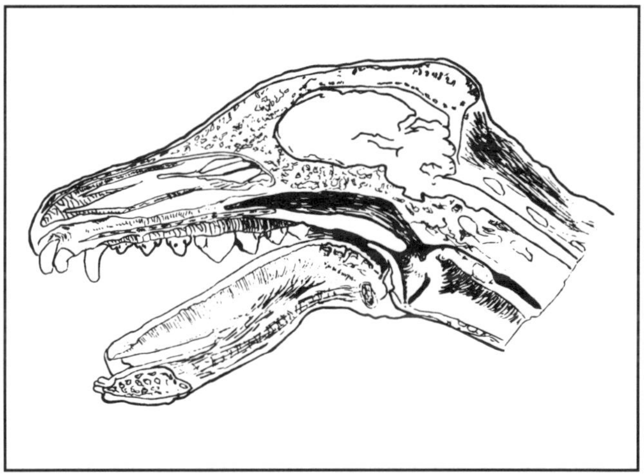

Fig. 3b. Section of head of collie dog showing how the large epiglottis is held in contact with the long soft palate.

there is food in the mouth. This is the stage of the so-called intranarial trachea.

With subsequent changes in the head and neck region, particularly in the extension of the neck and the greater mobility of the head, the role of the epiglottis increased markedly until it assumed the responsibility of sealing the airway between mouth and trachae. In almost all animals below man it makes contact with the soft palate lapping either the inferior (Fig. 3b) or superior (Fig. 3c) surface of the posterior margin of the velum. It maintains this

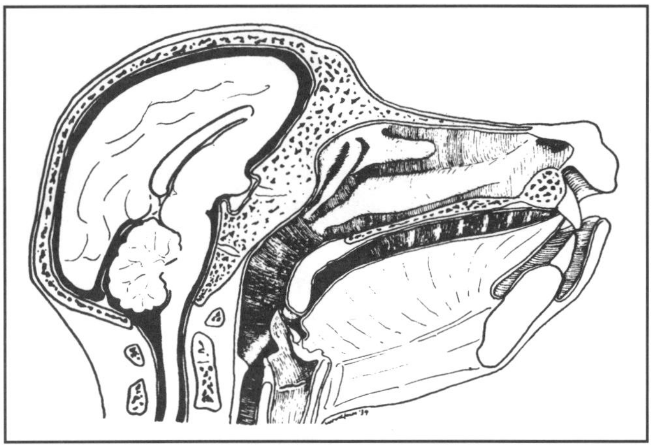

Fig. 3c. Well-developed epiglottis in primate holding down the upper surface of soft palate.

position at all times when the mouth is closed.

The habitual posture of various classes of animals

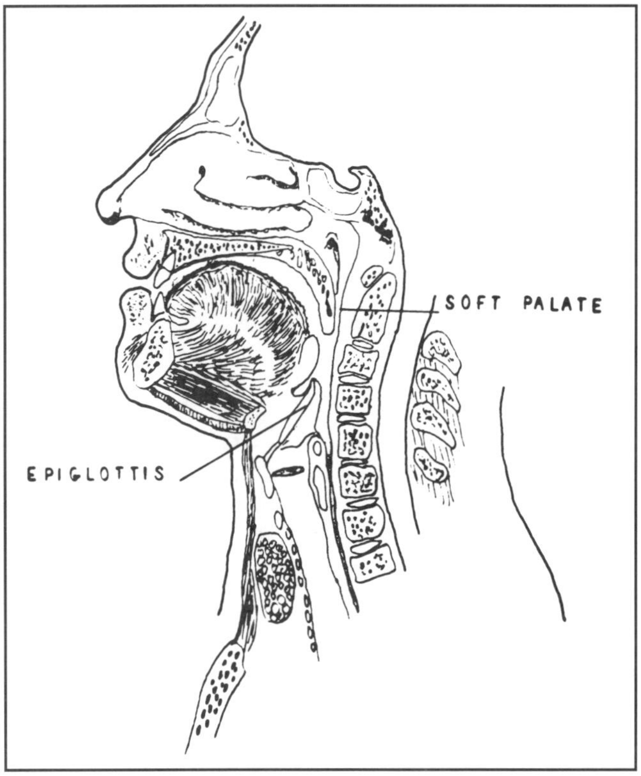

Fig. 3d. Vertical separation of soft palate and epiglottis in human.

has been shown to be closely correlated with laryngeal relations; the contact of the epiglottis with the soft palate, the direction of the opening of the glottis, and the mobility of the hyoid bone, all show progressive changes with each stage from the horizontally oriented tetrapod to the vertically-oriented, human biped.

The assumption of an habitual upright posture by humans required striking changes in laryngeal relations (Fig. 3d). The entire laryngeal complex, together with the hyoid bone from which it is suspended, is pulled down, making any contact between epiglottis and velum impossible. The soft palate now bears the responsibility for closing off the food channel from the nasopharynx. Such closure is necessary for deglutition, but according to Du Brul this change inadvertently made human speech possible, if not inevitable.

According to Wood-Jones, during deglutition in humans, the palatopharyngeus muscle acts the same as it has ever since the appearance of the aperture in the dorsal wall of the gut in the ganoid fishes and amphibia. In the early forms the aperture was surrounded by a sphincter as was previously described. In humans, the paired palatopharyngeus muscles originate in the soft palate and run backward and downward as the posterior pillars of the fauces. Passing with the superior constrictor of the pharynx to the posterior midline, they pinch together the walls of the muscular tube and close it from the nose and nasopharynx to form an upper pharyngeal seal.

The closure of the larynx might be thought of as occurring below; in fact there are two levels of closure within the larynx itself. The lower of these lies at the level of the vocal and vestibular cords which run between the anterior or vocal processes of the pyramidally-shaped arytenoid cartilages in back to the midline of the inner surface of the thyroid cartilage in front. The size of the triangular opening between their margins is controlled by the rotations of the arytenoid cartilages. Such movements, however, are probably not as important for sealing the glottis as for respiration and sound production.

The major actors in laryngeal closure seem to be the arytenoideus and the aryepiglottic muscles, as well as the epiglottis itself.

The arytenoideus obliquus muscles have their origins on the muscular processes of the arytenoid cartilages at the inferolateral extremities of the pyramids. They run medially and upward, crossing each other at the summits of the opposite cartilages. The aryepiglotti muscles run forward and upward around either side of the epiglottis from the anterior surface of the epiglottis. The function of this muscular complex is to tip the arytenoids

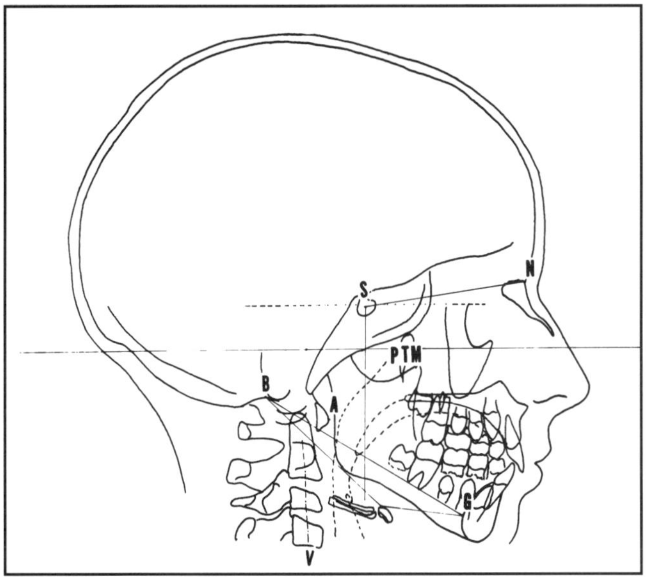

Fig. 3e. Tracing of landmarks.

forward and squeeze them together while puffing the epiglottis back at the level of its tubercle.

The anterior surface of the epiglottis is attached to the back of the tongue in the midline, and at its lateral borders as far down as the superior border of the thyroid cartilage. Hence, it is not free to bend backward in the manner of a hinged lid, as is frequently described. In the writer's view, closure of

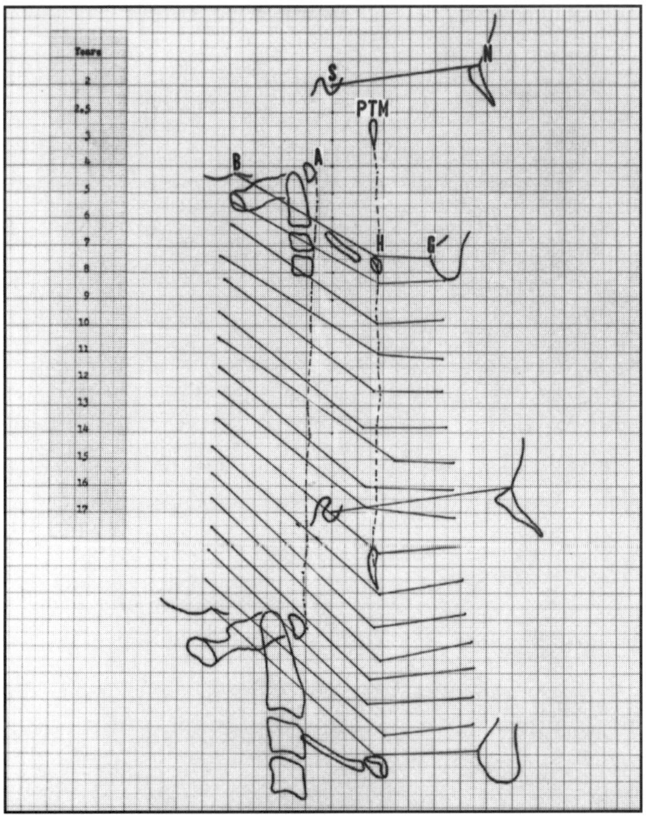

Fig. 3f. Changes in position and dimension of pharynx from two-to-18 years..

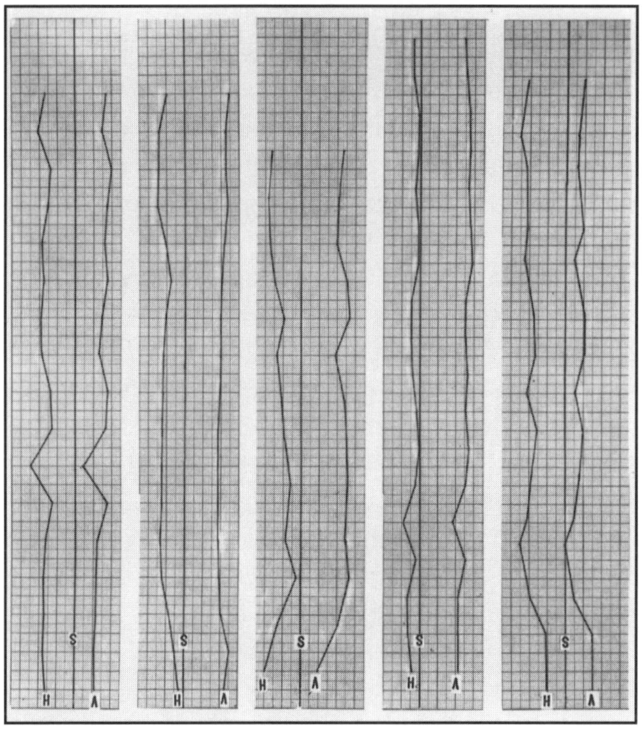

Fig. 3g. Individual variation of growth.

the larynx can be understood more logically through the following explanation.

The thyroepiglottic muscles, attached below to the inner surface of the thyroid cartilage close to the midline, run vertically to insert on the anterior surface of the epiglottis at the level of its tubercle. Since the epiglottis is fastened to the tongue, the contraction of these muscles would result in a backward buckling of the epiglottis at the level of the tubercle and a firmer sealing of its superior margin with the tongue. This is given greatly increased effectiveness by the aryepiglottic muscles which, it will be recalled, run upward and forward from the arytenoid cartilages to pass around the sides of the epiglottis and insert on its anterior surface.

Thus far, no mention has been made of two pairs of cartilage nodules, the cuneiform and the corniculates. These lie in the folds which enclose the aryepiglottic muscles and surmount the summits of the arytenoid cartilages at rest. When the arytenoid cartilages tip forward, these nodules are carried to a position that brings them into contact with the backwardly displaced tubercle. Thus it can be seen that the entrance from the pharynx into the larynx and trachea is guarded by a muscular sphincter, the margins of which are strengthened by cartilages tightly squeezed together.

The functions of respiration, deglutition, olfaction, and speech in man involve more than the opening and closing of valves between the gut and the airway. They require considerable movement of other organs or parts, changes in form, and in some cases adaptive changes in the position of parts in the interest of survival.

In human deglutition the extensive upward and backward rotary movement of the hyoid bone presses the bulk of the tongue successively against the hard palate, the soft palate, and the pharyngeal wall where the pharyngeal constrictors continue to propel the bolus downward in a peristaltic-like action. During this stage the ring of laryngeal cartilages are forcibly drawn together and literally buried in the base of the tongue to close the airway while the entry to the gut is opened.

Reflex Control of the Airway*

King in 1952 studied the growth of the pharynx in relation to certain cranial and vertebral bony points. Durzo in 1962, using the same method, sought to determine if there were any changes in position of the hyoid bone coincident with the vocal changes in males at adolescence. In an all male sample of serial cephalometric roentgenograms, he traced the details shown in Fig. 3e. He constructed the Frankfort horizontal and a vertical plane through "S" for references. Additional lines were drawn to "H," the highest point of the hyoid bone, from "B," the Bolton point, and from "G," the most posterior point on the silhouette of the symphysis of the mandible. The last point represented the genial tubercles. Two resulting lines represented the posterior and anterior suprahyoid muscles respectively. "A" represented the most anterior point on the axis (Fig. 3f). Because the flexions of the cervical vertebrae had occurred during exposure of some of the cephalograms, points in "B" and in "H" did not follow straight downward courses parallel with that from "S" but, significantly, remained parallel to each other (Fig. 3g).

The anterior posterior dimension of the airway remained unchanged from three to 17 years as determined by measurements made at the shortest distance between the hyoid point and the vertebrae. Failure of the mandible to move downward and forward with growth in one subject suffering an arrest of condylar development was shown to maintain her original airway dimension by a gradual increase of the tensions of the anterior hyoid muscles (Fig. 3h). This seems to indicate to us that the dimension of the airway is controlled by reflex.

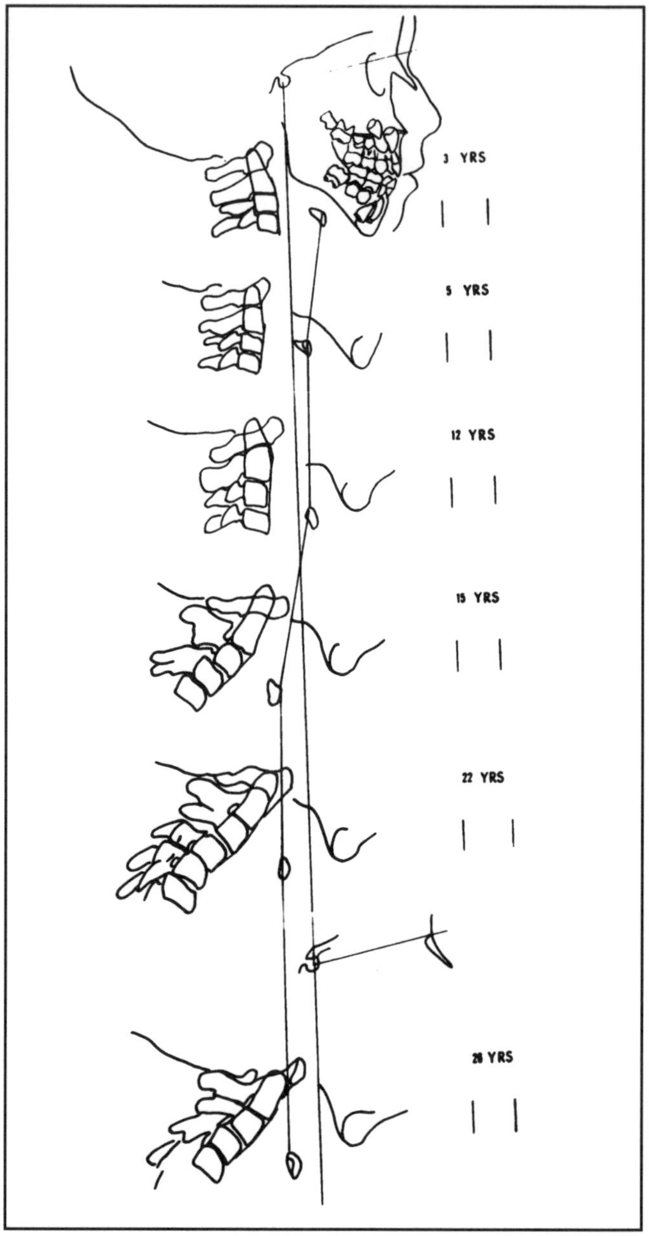

Fig. 3h. Three-to-26 years.

*See Appendix II: Endnotes.

Reading list:

Durzo, Carmine. *Growth behavior of the Hyoid bone: a serial x-ray study.* Thesis (MS in orthodontia), University of Illinois, 1961.

Negus, V.E. *The Comparative Anatomy and Physiology of the Larynx.* London: Heinemann Medical Books Ltd., 1949.

4. Laryngeo-Pharyngeal Mechanism

Had air-breathing not been an essential requirement of terrestial existence, the pharynx would probably have remained a simple structure. One cannot imagine the need for more than a funnel-like structure with contractile walls to convey the contents of the mouth to the gut. Also, had the air intake remained ventral to the gut, as are the gills of fishes, the food ingesting and air procuring systems could have remained separate and relatively independent. It was apparently the demands of another of the special senses, olfaction, that made necessary certain changes in the relationship of the two systems.

In a water environment, both oxygen and odors have been derived from that medium by different anatomical routes. While oxygen was abstracted by the gills, odors were detected in a stream of water which entered the head above the mouth, circulated over a specialized area of the brain, and was discharged through more posterior apertures. This primitive means of detecting food and enemies served until the energy demand of the animal made increased oxygen intake essential. This need was met by the development of the internal lung.

There were other adaptations that permitted humans to attain an upright posture and simultaneously to gain the advantage of articular speech. This is understandable on the following basis: in a four-footed animal the food and air channels travel together, suspended in a nearly horizontal course to the thorax, whereas in the erect biped both tubes must be flexed at the junction of the head and body. Much of the respiratory channel is protected by firm walls—above by the bone of the nose, and below by the larynx and trachea. Above the two is the pharynx, a soft tissue structure which must serve both channels. Except for very short intervals the airway must be kept open, but the food channel must be distended only while food is being swallowed.

In other mammals, the hyoid bone and its musculature are concerned largely with respiration and deglutition, but in humans it also plays a critical role in the maintenance of their upright posture. The anterior members of the suprahyoid group of muscles, geniohyoid and mylohyoid, not only constitute the most superior link in the anterior chain of postural muscles, but maintain the patency of the airway by holding the entire laryngeal mechanism forward while doing so.

If the human airway is compared to a hose, one can readily imagine that its lumen could be affected at different levels along its course. The first such level lies within the bony nose where inflammatory swelling of the mucous membrane of the conchae, exostoses, or deviations of the septum may serve to impede the flow of air.

The next level of possible interference is the epipharynx, or that part of the pharynx behind the nose. Here the openings from the nose, the posterior nares, are occasionally undersized. More frequently, however, obstructions in the form of lymphoid tissue, the adenoid, is present in the form of a large swelling of the roof and posterior wall of the pharynx. These may be gross enough to contact the soft palate and completely close the airway above the level of the palate. Under such circumstances, the child has no recourse but to breathe through the mouth.

At a slightly lower level on both sides of the base of the tongue lie the faucial tonsils, twin masses of lymphoid tissue which lie lingually to the rami of the mandible between the anterior and posterior pillars of the fauces. The tonsils, adenoids, the thymus, and the tongue all are large at birth and continue to increase in size until the beginning of adolescence, after which they tend to shrink quite rapidly.

The tongue at birth completely fills the mouth and flows out over the margins of the jaws. Any hypertrophy of the organ during this period poses threats to the infants respiration and deglutition. The first is compensated by mouth-breathing, but the act of swallowing requires that the mouth be closed. Closure forces the tongue back sufficiently to excite the gag reflex, causing regurgitation. This makes feeding very difficult.

Deglutition

The necessity of maintaining an adequate airway

almost continuously in all air-breathing animals is evidenced by the multitude of adaptations encountered in any survey of the function of deglutition in the various animal forms. Such adaptations indicate that they serve the wide variety of demands made upon them by variations in the nature of food available to each and in the method of preparation of the food intraorally (teeth, tongue, lips, cheeks, jaws and jaw joint, head skeleton, and muscles of mastication and neck). In addition to these are the demands for the maintenance of olfaction and those imposed by gravity, which have resulted from the gradual change from horizontal to upright posture. All of these and more are reflected in the complex act of swallowing. The reader interested in the many fascinating ramifications of these matters is referred to the writings of Negus and Bosma. Here we shall be concerned only with the act of deglutition in the human species.

Humans are unique in that their upright posture has been made possible partly by the enlistment of their hyoid musculature into the ventral chain of muscles, counteracting those of the antigravitational system. This has been an accommodation in the change in the craniovertebral relation associated with deflection of both air and food channels. Further adaptations have brought the hyoid bone to such a low level in the neck that the epiglottis can no longer make contact with the soft palate. This necessitates more extensive movements of the hyoid bone and associated structures during swallowing, but at the same time has made articulated speech possible, indeed almost inevitable, according to Du Brul.

The preparatory stage of deglutition in the case of non-fluid food consists of a gathering of the food on the upper surface of the more anterior portion of the tongue ahead of the area where it makes contact with the hard palate. The food is moved backward on the tongue toward the fauces by a peristaltic wave-like alteration of the shape of the tongue as the teeth are brought together. Simultaneously with this there is a tensing of the floor of the mouth, which transforms the mylohyoid muscle from a trough-like structure to an elevated flat surface. This aids in elevating the tongue.

Until this time events can be thought of as being voluntary, but now they become involuntary. Owing to the rapidity of action and the difficulty of direct observation, the exact sequence of events during the following stages is not universally agreed upon, but the following description seems to be the most plausible integration of the information presently available.

Immediately prior to the act of swallowing, the hyoid bone is partially elevated. This posture of the hyoid is associated with the cessation of intraoral manipulation and of breathing. As the tongue is elevated by the styloglossus, the palate is depressed to meet it by the palatoglossus. At this stage, the bolus has been brought to a position on the posterior aspect of the tongue and against the hard palate above, tapering into the convergence of the tongue and the soft palate.

Radiological studies show that the bolus is then carried from the dorsum of the tongue almost vertically downward between the tongue and the diagonal walls formed as the medial edges of the palatopharyngeal muscles are straightened by tension and brought into apposition with each other. This muscular structure forms the palatopharyngeal partition, which now constitutes a new posterior wall of the oral pharynx effectively separating the food and air channels.

As the bolus moves downward toward the epiglottis, reflexes set a number of actions in motion. The hyoid bone is raised to its maximum level and carried backward while the tongue rolls back over it. Coincidentally, the muscular pharynx is raised and dilated by its extrinsic muscles, principally the stylopharyngeus, in what Negus has called an "engulfing action." The hyoid is literally buried in the base of the tongue by the hyoglossus while the larynx is carried to its highest level. This crushing together of tongue, hyoid bone, and larynx combines with the action of the extrinsic muscles of the larynx to close the glottis against the ingress of food into the trachea.

The study of the progress of a radiopaque bolus by cinefluoroscopy indicates that the act of swallowing is not a smooth, even course of events; nor is it the same in all individuals. It even varies with the consistency of the food being swallowed; fluids are swallowed differently than firmer foods. In almost all cases, however, the tongue acts as the propelling agent to thrust the bolus from the mouth into the pharynx. On arrival there, the constrictors take over with a reflex peristaltic action as the pharynx settles down to its resting level.

During the course of these happenings, the hyoid bone and larynx are jerked forward together underneath the tongue, which opens the pharynx anteriorly into the upper end of the esophagus. When this sudden ventral movement is viewed by cineflourscopy, it gives the impression of "jerking the rug" from under the bolus.

During this brief but almost violent (convulsive?) swallowing episode, the mandible is stabilized by compensating contractions of its own muscular suspension system, which usually maintains a light occlusal contact of upper and lower teeth. Hardly a muscle in the entire craniofacial complex escapes some measure of participation in this contraction wave which accompanies the swallowing act.

Although the above description of human deglutition finds the majority of writers in general agreement with that of Majendie (1822), modern studies have revealed additional ramification of the swallow. This has come about by the establishment of centers for the treatment of cleft palate and speech disorders in which the value of a multidisciplinary approach has been demonstrated. Whereas the surgeon has previously been the sole arbiter of the management of cleft palate cases, it was found that better results were attained from a consensus of a team which also included the pediatrician, the orthodontist, and the speech therapist. Each of these brought methods and findings of studies from his own field.

One of the first examples of such cross fertilization was the application of longitudinal growth studies by means of roentgenographic cephalometry. Besides furnishing the means to follow the results of surgical intervention on the individual, it allowed comparisons to be made with normal samples already available at several centers where growth studies were being conducted. The cleft palate center at the University of Illinois was established under the supervision of Pruzansky, himself an orthodontist already conditioned in the multidisciplinary approach. With the aid of the Department of Anesthesiology, a method for the safe sedation of infants was developed and the taking of serial impressions and cephalograms was begun.

Subtelny described the method he had developed to measure the distance between the medial pterygoid lamina from laminagrams taken according to Brader's technique, and demonstrated greater than normal widths in unoperated cleft-palate cleft-lip children. This appeared to be due to the separation of the two maxillae by outward pull of the tensor veli palatinus muscles principally when the continuity of the labiobuccal musculature was broken. This finding led rapidly to a change in the order of surgical procedures, the lip now being operated on in early infancy and the palatalal closure being deferred until all possible natural growth closure had occurred. Indeed, obturation came to be preferred over extensive surgery in cases with wide persistent palatal clefts (Fig. 4a).

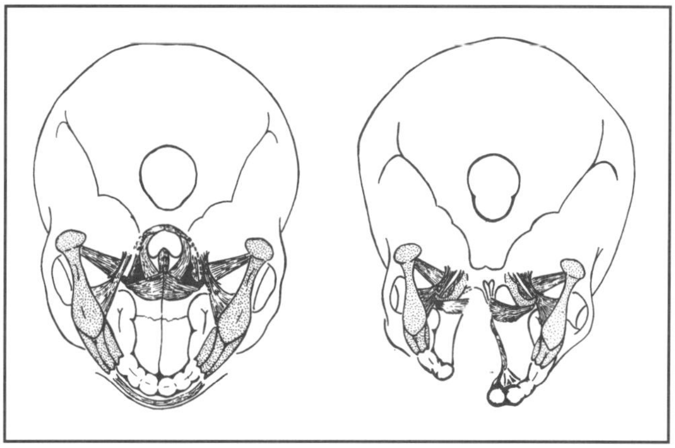

Fig. 4a. Tracing of normal (left) and cleft (right) palates.

Deglutition has been held to be implicated in many conditions other than the transfer to the pharynx and in speech. Because the teeth are brought into occlusion during swallowing, it has been believed that deglutition aids to guide them

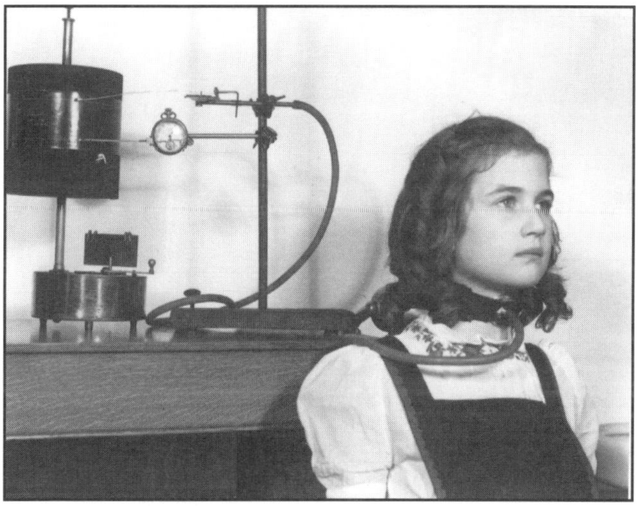

Fig. 4b. Apparatus to count frequency of swallowing.

into interdigitation and to maintain them there. It has been held to contribute to deep bite through depression of the posterior teeth caused and maintained by excessive contacting of the teeth.

Kincaid designed an apparatus to count the frequency of swallows in 50 individuals, 21 boys and 29 girls between nine and 14 years of age. Nineteen were Class I malocclusions, 22 were Class II, Div. I, and nine were Class II, Div. 2. Each individual was tested at two separate sittings of one half hour each. It was found that deglutition in the individual showed a tendency to follow a fairly constant rate, but the rate among the members of the sample ranged from 10 to 138 an hour.

Reading list:

Kincaid, Robert Myron. *The frequency of deglutition in man; its relationship to overbite.* Thesis (MS in orthodontia), University of Illinois, 1949.

Subtelny, Jacob Daniel. *Width of the Nasopharynx and Related Anatomical Structures in Normal and Unoperated Cleft Palate Children.* Thesis (MS in orthodontia), University of Illinois, 1953.

5.
Respiration

During quiet respiration, the structures of the cheeks, lips, soft palate, tongue, fauces, pharynx, and larynx are in a state of equilibrium, with the muscles in resting tonus. All functional movements start from this resting relationship, so any discussion of function must begin with a view of the relationships of parts that exist in that state.

The Tongue

The tongue is almost completely composed of and controlled by musculature. Its shape is adjusted by its intrinsic muscles which, running in three planes of space, determine its form at any given instant. At rest it fills the mouth almost completely, contacting the hard and soft palates and the lingual surfaces of the teeth. It is maintained in this position by extrinsic muscles that run to it from skeletal points on the cranium, mandible, and hyoid bone. Indeed, the hyoid bone can be considered the base from which the tongue operates, and since this bone is similarly suspended from many of the same directions, the two may be considered almost as a unit.

From the styloid process of the temporal bone the styloglossus and stylohyoid muscles run downward, forward, and somewhat medially to both tongue and hyoid bone. These are both long, spindly muscles affording a large range of movement in an upward and backward direction.

Anteroposterior positioning is controlled from the inner surface of the mandible at the midline by the geniohyoglossus and, only slightly lateral to this, the geniohyoid muscles. These act in some measure to counterbalance the styloglossus and stylohyoideus muscles. Vertical positioning of the base of the tongue also is influenced in a large measure by the palatoglossus and hyoglossus muscles.

From all this, it can be realized that the tongue and the hyoid bone are wholly suspended in space, with their positions determined from two lateral points posteriorly and a single midline point anteriorly. This imparts a "centering" tendency that can be disturbed only by an unnatural placement of the points of suspension, as in skeletal asymmetry, or abnormalities of the neuromuscular system.

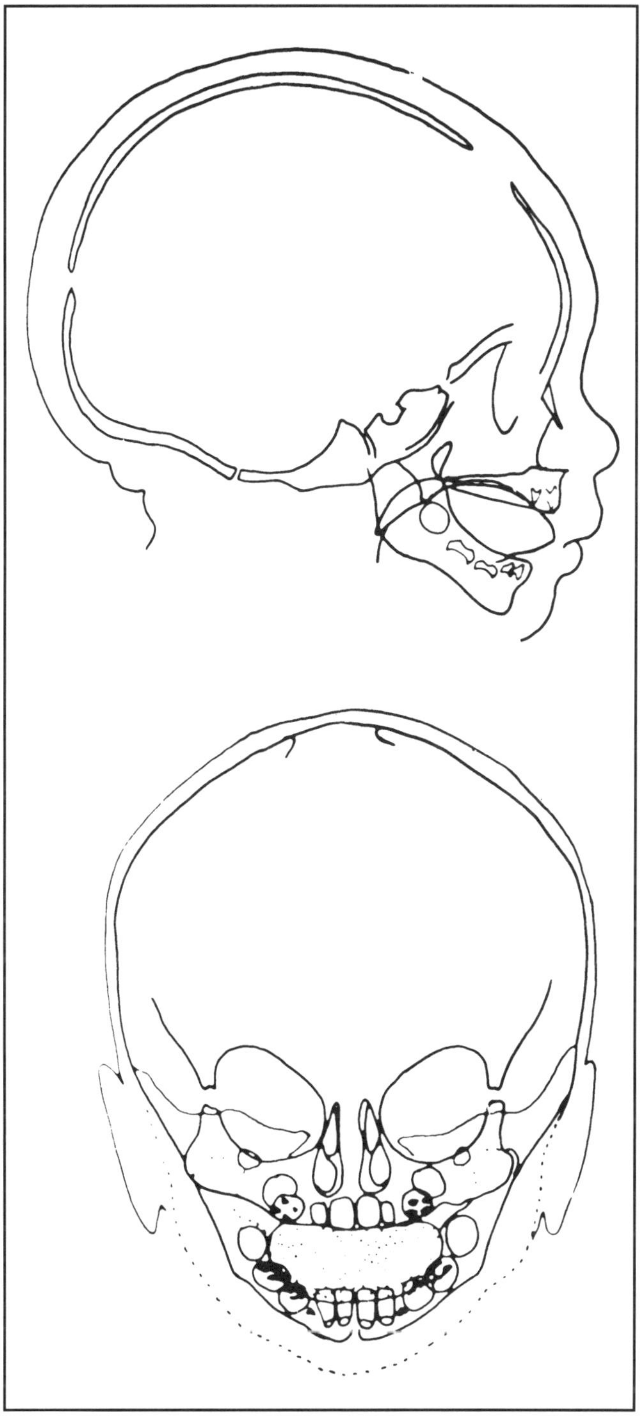

Fig. 5a. Position of the tongue in a newborn.

The Soft Palate

This structure can be understood if one imagines a sheet or aponeurosis attached to the posterior border of the hard palate from side to side, with muscles running to it from above and below. The muscles act to cause the soft palate to close the airway during deglutition and speech. In its habitual position, the concave anterior surface rests upon the base of the tongue while the convex posterior surface forms the anterior wall of the pharynx. At rest it is separated from the posterior pharyngeal wall by an interval of about a quarter of an inch, which forms the airway.

During deglutition and phonation of vowel sounds, the nasopharynx is closed by two pairs of muscles which run to the soft palate from above.

One of these, the tensor veli palatini, takes extensive origin from the spinous processes of the great wings of the sphenoid, the cartilagenous auditory tubes, and the scaphoid fossa at the roots of the medial pterygoid plate. The fibers converge as they run down the medial pterygoid plates and form tendons which run around the hamuli. Direction is thus changed from vertical to horizontal. These muscles might be thought of as piercing the lateral walls of the pharynx, although they actually run between the superior and middle constrictors. Leaving the hamulus, the fibers of the tendons intermingle with those of the palatine aponuerosis. The contraction of the vertical muscular portion tenses the horizontal fibrous part, making it firm and raising it into contact with the posterior pharyngeal wall.

The other pair of muscles, namely the levators veli palatini, arise from the undersurface of the tip of the petrous part of the temporal bone and adjacent auditory tubes and enter the pharynx over the superior margin of the superior constrictor. They run downward and medialward to mingle with fibers from the opposite side and of the aponuerosis in the area of the midline. The action of this muscle raises the middle of the soft palate so that it extends the dome of the hard palate to the posterior pharyngeal wall.

The muscles that antagonize the levators and contribute to the position of the soft palate at rest are the palatoglossus and the palatopharyngeus.

The palatoglossus arises from the anterior surface of the soft palate where it joins with its fellow of the opposite side. It curves laterally and downward to mingle with the fibers of the side of the tongue spreading over the dorsum and deeper, intermingling with the transverse fibers. Thus, with the tongue moving back during deglutition, the palatoglossus acts as a barrier against the return of food into the mouth.

The palatopharyngeus arises by two heads in the palate, where it is divided by the levator into two fasciculi. The anterior of these joins its opposite member at the midline and from here arches backward and downward, spreading along the side of the pharynx. The most anterior fibers mingle with those of the stylopharyngeus to insert into the posterior border of the thyroid cartilage, and its posterior fibers join those of its opposite member at the posterior midline of the pharynx. According to Wood-Jones, the palatopharyngeus muscle is the modern form of the palatal sphincter, which held the intranarial trachae in place in early air-breathing forms. This same author traces the musculus uvula back to a cluster of lubricuating glands situated at the midline of the anterior border of the sphincter.

The Pharynx

The intrinsic structures of the pharynx are made up of the superior, middle, and inferior constrictor muscles, fasciae, and membranes. The pharynx hangs in the manner of an oriole's nest behind the face and just anterior to the cervical part of the vertebral column.

In back the pharynx is attached to the precervical fascia by a median fibrous raphe, which is attached above to the pharyngeal tubercle on the basilar part of the occipital bone. Thus, the posterior wall of the pharynx is relatively fixed, being movable only with the movement of the vertebrae to which it is attached. The front part of the pharynx is quite different, in that it provides the openings for the nasal and oral cavities as well as the esophagus and larynx.

The lateral walls of the pharynx are formed largely by the constrictors. The superior takes its anterior attachment from the posterior margin of the medial pterygoid lamina, beginning at the process tubarius. This also is the point for entrance of the medial end of the cartilagenous auditory tube into the nasopharynx. From this point, the superior constrictor continues down to attach to the hamulus and to the fibrous raphe, which runs from the hamulus to the end of the mylohyoid line on the lingual side of the mandible. The superior margin of the muscle follows an arched course from the process tubarius backward and upward to the pharyngeal tubercle. It is over this superior margin that the levator veli palatini travels from the tip of the petrous part of the temporal bone to reach the soft palate. The space between the superior margin of the muscle and the base of the skull, known as the sinus of Morgagny, is closed by the pharyngeal aponeurosis, which constitutes the domed roof of the naso or epipharynx.

The middle constrictor is closely associated with the hyoid bone. It takes its anterior attachment from the entire superior surface of the greater and lesser cornua of that bone and continues up for a short distance on the stylohyoid ligament. Its superior fibers run upward as they encircle the pharyngeal space, overlapping the superior constrictor and joining its own fellow of the opposite side at the median raphe. The inferior fibers run downward as they curve backward to the raphe and are lapped by the inferior constrictor.

Before considering the inferior constrictor, the relation between the hyoid bone and thyroid cartilage should be reviewed. The two are connected by the hyothyroid membrane, a sheet of fibroelastic tissue which is attached below to the entire upper border of the thyroid cartilage and to the anterior surfaces of its superior cornua. Passing upward within the hyoid bone and its greater cornua, it inserts on the superior margin from end to end. At the midline in front the membrane is thickened into the middle hyothyroid ligament. On each side in back a similar thickening forms the lateral hyothyroid ligaments, which join the hyoid with the thyroid cornua. This arrangement precludes any but very small movements in limited directions between the hyoid bone and the larynx. In all major movements of the hyoid bone, the larynx must follow.

The inferior is the heaviest of the constrictors. It arises from the sides of the cricoid and thyroid cartilages along a line that extends from the inferior border of the cricoid to the superior border of the thyroid. From here the superior fibers course upward and backward, overlapping the middle constrictor and inserting into the median raphe. The inferior fibers run horizontally backward and are continuous with the circular fibers of the esophagus. Hence it is apparent that the pharynx is completed in front by the tongue, epiglottis, and larynx (Fig. 5b).

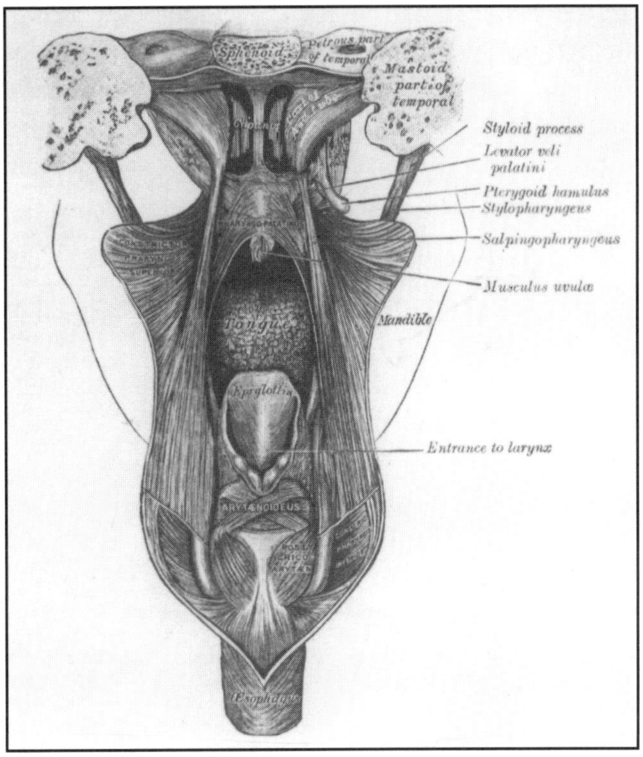

Fig. 5b. Muscles of pharynx as seen from posterior.

Pharyngeal function is further controlled by three pairs of extrinsic muscles—the stylopharyngeus, salpingopharyngeus, and palatopharyngeus. The last have already been described with the soft palate.

The stylopharyngeus is the chief muscle of suspension and movement of the pharynx. It is a long, slender muscle taking its insertion from the base of the styloid process and passing downward and slightly medially along the side of the pharynx between the superior and middle constrictors to spread out and intermingle with the fibers of the palatopharyngeus. Both send fibers to the posterior border of the thyroid cartilage.

The salpingopharyngeus arises from the inferior part of the auditory tube near its orifice and passes downward to blend with the posterior fasciculus of the palatopharyngeus. The stylopharyngeus elevates and widens the pharynx during deglutition while the salpingopharyngeus simultaneously controls the cartilaginous orifice of the auditory tube. At rest, the patency of this orifice is maintained by a firm prominence, the torus. It is closed by the salpingopharyngeus during swallowing.

The orifice may be partially or completely blocked by lymphoid tissue (adenoid or pharyngeal tonsil) or by secretions from the nose during severe head colds or similar infections. Sudden increases in air pressure as in a sudden descent in airplanes or elevators is frequently accompanied by closure and earache. Swallowing or wide opening of the mouth as in yawning usually will be sufficient to open the orifice and reestablish the balance of air pressure on the tympanum of the middle ear.

6.
The Evolution of Tooth Form

Accompanying the demand for increased amounts of oxygen went adaptations in the food procuring mechanism as well as increased efficiency of the rest of the digestive system. Only recently has the latter come to be subjected to critical study, but the teeth, being frequently preserved because of their calcified nature, have been susceptible to such study for a long time. As a result there is a large amount of evidence available to explain their evolution.

The forerunners of the teeth, the placoid scales, first arose as shagreen on the covering of the body. From here they invaded the stomodeum, advancing over its margins until they are thought to have lined it and even extended part way down the gut. Evidence for this lies in presence of teeth on the palatine and vomerine bones of many fish and reptiles. These animals have spines, which aid in forcing living prey down the alimentary tract.

In those forms, which are thought to lie on the stem which advances to higher levels, the precursors of the teeth were limited to the margins of the jaws. They increased in height and took on slight curvatures, and from the earliest forms showed an arrangement in which the teeth of the lower jaw were received within those of the upper and there was an alternation, so that the teeth of one jaw closed opposite to the space between two teeth of the other jaw.

These early teeth were apparently nothing more than mounds of an epithelium, the summits of which were calcified. As they increased in height and were subject to more strenuous function, the calcified portion took on greater and greater hardness, which gradually resulted in the very specialized tissue enamel. This tissue in turn led to another tissue to support it (dentine), which was derived from the underlying mesenchyme. (Enamel still has the specialized property of calling forth dentine, as witnessed by the formation of dentine in apposition to it when transplanted into any mesenchymal environment in the body)

These early teeth, like all those succeeding them, were tools devoted to the grasping of food, and the food of early forms was largely other living forms. As they increased in size their usefulness was determined by the firmness with which they were fastened to the jaws. Thus, here accompanied their growth a gradual modification of their attachment. Beginning with a fibrous union there evolved a direct ankylosis with another newly derived tissue, bone, which had developed from the cartilage beneath them.

From the very beginning teeth have shown the conical pattern, but in the early forms and lower forms today these cones are independent of each other. Eventually there arose multicuspid teeth, and the manner in which this occurred has been debated for many years. For the purposes of these studies it will suffice to mention the various theories that have been advanced, and to deal more fully with the one that is supported by the best evidence.

The earliest theory is that known as "concrescence," suggested by Kenthal and Rose. This theory held that as the jaws shortened, the teeth were crowded together and a coalescence of several simple cusps occurred. In view of what is known today about the manner in which teeth develop embryologically, this seems untenable. True, a fusion of teeth is occasionally seen, but this is not in the nature of cusp addition.

Another theory held that the movements of the jaw dictated where cusps would arise and that the form of the glenoid fossa was largely responsible. This would make it appear that teeth could be squeezed into a form by function, which is obviously impossible. Also, it should be pointed out that teeth antedated the joint by millions of years.

Cope advanced the idea that cusps arose at the points of greatest wear. This argument falls down when it is considered that one tooth would receive the same amount of wear as its antagonist, hence cusp must meet cusp instead of cusp meeting fossa.

The cingulum theory (Marett Times) is supported best by evidence. The cingulum is a ridge which surrounds the neck of a tooth. It is a very ancient structure, as all primitive teeth exhibit it, and it was probably a means of additional anchorage for them. By its disappearance in some parts and its elevation in others, the form of a tooth could be profoundly altered. This theory is supported by the Growth Gradient Theory of Schour, which demonstrates strikingly how secondary growth centers may appear in the tooth germs of modern humans and lead to additional cusps in a matter of a few generations. This is shown in the cusp of Carabelli on the palatal side of the upper first permanent molar, which is a familial trait.

But regardless of how the cusps arose there eventually appeared a tricuspid tooth. It exhibited three cones in a line, a large middle one (protocone), a smaller anterior one (paracone), and a smaller posterior one (metacone). These teeth were arranged in a definite manner, with those of the upper jaw overhanging those of the lower and alternating with each other. Such teeth, obviously, had little advantage over the simple cones they replaced, in that they could merely grasp prey (Fig. 6a).

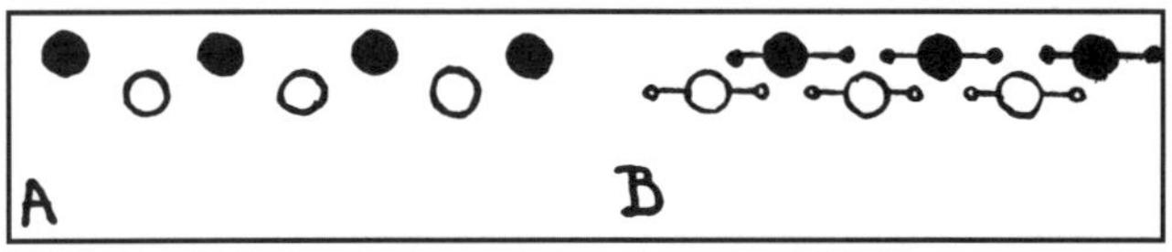

Fig. 6a. Occlusal view of relationship between upper and lower teeth. A, as it is in dentitions with simple conical teeth; B, as it is in triconodont teeth.

The next modification witnessed the arrangement of the cusps in the form of a triangle or triad with the larger cusp of the upper at the apex and situated on the palatal side. The triangle of the lower presented its principal cusp toward the buccal side and, since the upper and lower teeth alternated, there was now interdigitation but still no occlusion (Fig. 6b, 6c).

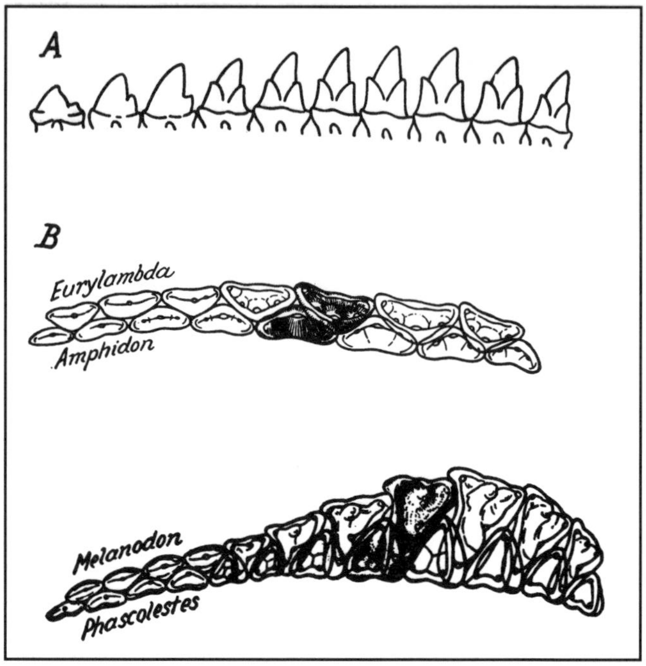

Fig. 6b.

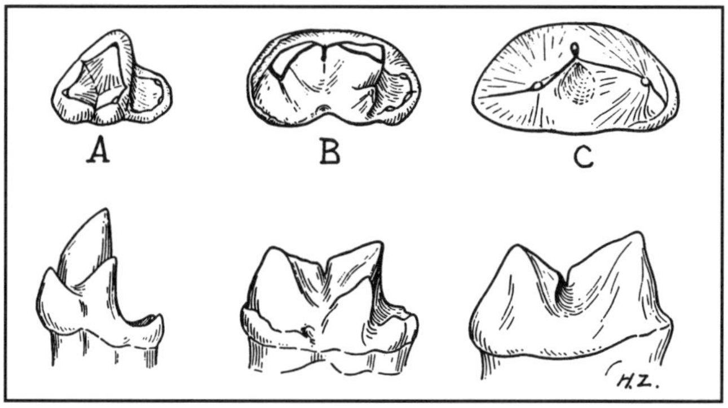

Fig 6c. Structural evolution of lower shearing tooth.

From the earlier forms, i.e., those which exhibited the three cusps in a line, there emerged teeth capable of shearing flesh. This came about through the appearance of ridges, which connected the cusps accompanied by a buccolingual flattening of the cusps themselves. In this manner sharp, notched edges could be made to work against each other in the manner of shears. The mechanics of this action will be dealt with later.

In those forms which developed the triangular teeth which interlocked with each other, there developed a fourth cone (hypocone). This arose from the posterior marginal ridge and came to be received in the fossa formed by the three cusps of the tooth of the opposite jaw. Now, for the first time, there was an arrangement that could be called occlusion. Teeth now struck each other as the jaws were closed, and the path was open for the herbivorous and omnivorous dentitions.

It seems more logical to believe that the omnivorous pattern antedated the herbivorous than vice versa on the basis of fossil evidence. The teeth of the mastodon, forerunner of the modern elephant, were large, block-shaped, and surmounted by moderate height enamel-covered cones connected by and over the cusps. The diet, which carried large amounts of earth with it, led to rapid wear which soon resulted in exposure of the underlying dentine. Although this arrangement presented an occlusal surface admirably adapted to the milling of plant fibers, there was not sufficient enamel to prevent excessive wear. Further adaptation in the matter of tooth formation met this need in the following manner.

All teeth exhibit the simple cone form in the earliest stages of formation; this cone is delineated by the dento-enamel junction. On the outside of this junction enamel will be formed, and in apposition to it on the inside dentine will appear.

Now if one imagines this structure as a finger of a glove and then further visualizes the result of pushing the tip of the finger up inside of it with a small instrument, a clear picture of the mode of formation of herbivorous teeth can be gained. Not only would the entire outer surface be covered with enamel, but the pressed-in portion would be lined with enamel. The condition of *dens in dentis*, seen occasionally in the human, is a striking example of this phenomenon. Here it is an anomaly, but let us see how it works to great advantage in the animal living on plant food. The molar of the horse is a good model (Fig. 6d).

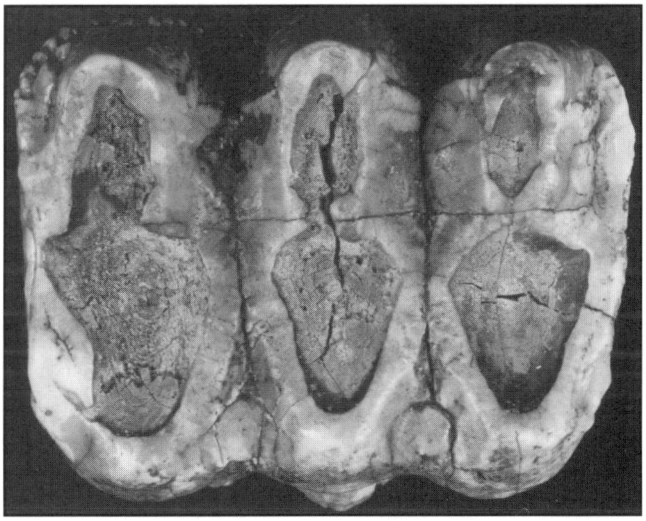

Fig. 6d. Pattern of wear on herbivorous molars.

When this tooth erupts it may be covered with cementum, and the cavity formed by the infolding of the enamel organ is filled with this tissue. No evidence of this is apparent at first, but as the tooth is worn there appears a band of enamel which parallels the outline of the tooth when viewed from the incisal aspect. This enamel ring surrounds a field of cementum.

With further wear, the enamel ring becomes two concentric rings and between them appears the dentine. The outer ring will remain with the outline of the tooth while the inner ring becomes progressively smaller since the folded-in enamel organ tapers as it goes apically. This pattern of the inner ring of the horse incisor is known as the "mark" and is an accurate gauge of the physiological age of the animal. Hence the implied discourtesy of "looking a gift horse in the mouth."

In the buccal teeth of the herbivorous animals the process of tooth formation is the same as that just described, but the foldings of the enamel organ are more numerous. They may occur on any surface—occlusal, buccal, or lingual—and follow any course. This gives rise to very complicated patterns of wear, but such patterns are distinct for each species. How do they serve the grazing animal?

Since wear is suffered by the entire occlusal surface of the tooth, three tissues of different indices of wear are exposed. Enamel, being the hardest, wears least and hence presents ridges that stand at greater height than the rest. The next hardest tissue is dentine, and it stands at a slightly lower lever. Cementum, being the softest, wears the fastest and lies the lowest. Thus, the teeth become admirably adapted for shredding and are kept efficient by the animal's side-to-side function. Even the hardest tissue, enamel, is not permitted to become smooth since its prisms are arranged horizontally and hence, subject to chipping. This exposes new sharp edges in the same manner that the breaking off of crystals keeps a carborundum stone efficient.

Since all teeth, like tools, are subject to a wearing process or to accident, it is interesting to note that all are endowed with some sort of mechanism for adjustment to this wear so that their efficiency is maintained throughout life. Mention has already been made of this mechanism in the most primitive forms where, if a tooth is torn out, another forms.

In the carnivorous animals this adjustment appears to reside in the bone of the jaws or, more correctly perhaps, in the periodontal membrane. The teeth of these animals pass each other in their strictly vertical function, and hence wear would occur on the buccal surfaces of the lower teeth and the palatal surfaces of the upper. Such wear is minimal because of the very hard enamel of these animals as well as their great efficiency in shearing. But any wear that *did* occur would have to be adjusted to either by a greater lateral shift of the mandible or by a bodily movement of the mandibular teeth in a buccal direction or a palatal movement of those of the maxilla. To determine which it was, the following experiment was performed.

The canine and carnassial teeth of cats were ground—the lowers on the buccal, the uppers on the lingual sides—and measurements were made between the corresponding teeth of the two sides. Naturally, the grinding had decreased the distance between the lowers and increased that between the uppers. After a short interval of days the measurements were repeated, and they were found to be the same as before the grinding. It thus appears that the teeth of this type of animal are adjusted by some phenomenon that causes the lower to try to move buccally and the upper lingually.

A different type of adjustment is found in the plant-fiber eaters. Their wear is largely on the occlusal surface so that if it were not adjusted there would occur a closing of the bite. These teeth enjoy perpetual eruption. Although completely formed early in life they are very tall and they erupt as fast as their occlusal surfaces wear. But the incisor of the rodent exhibits the most active response to wear; indeed if these animals do not wear their teeth, they are killed by them.

The purest type of rodent possesses only four incisors, two above and two below. The uppers arise anterior to the buccal teeth, follow an arc through the front of the maxilla, converging toward each other and emerging in front where they touch interproximally. The lowers arise near the posterior border of the ramus, follow a larger arc which lies close to the lower border of the mandible, converge toward the midline, and touch each other interproximally after they emerge at the front of the mouth.

These teeth are hard-working tools. They have no role in the preparing of food for digestion; they are designed to permit the animal to *get at* his food. They can fell trees (beaver) or gnaw through a lead pipe (rat). To do this they must constantly be sharpened, which leads to rapid wear. To compensate for this wear they grow continuously at their forming ends. They are known as teeth of perpetual growth, in contradistinction to teeth of perpetual succession or teeth of perpetual eruption described above (Fig. 6e).

But the pattern of wear of the rodent incisor tells us much more than the fact that it grows continually. When these teeth first form they exhibit the

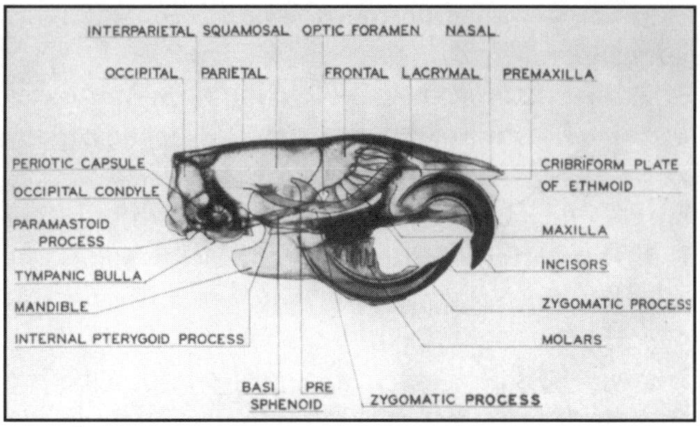

Fig. 6e. Rodent dentition occluding on molars.

cone design basic to all teeth, but function quickly changes this. Indeed, their functional design is well established before they are born because they begin to sharpen their teeth before this. They must continue this activity as long as they live, as witness the motion of the snout even when the animal is not feeding.

An examination of the form of the working area of these teeth as seen from the side requires explanation. We note immediately that if they were approximated, they could meet only at their very thin labial edges. Behind these edges both present concave surfaces, whereas one might expect they would be concentric to each other—one concave, the other convex. More careful scrutiny of their

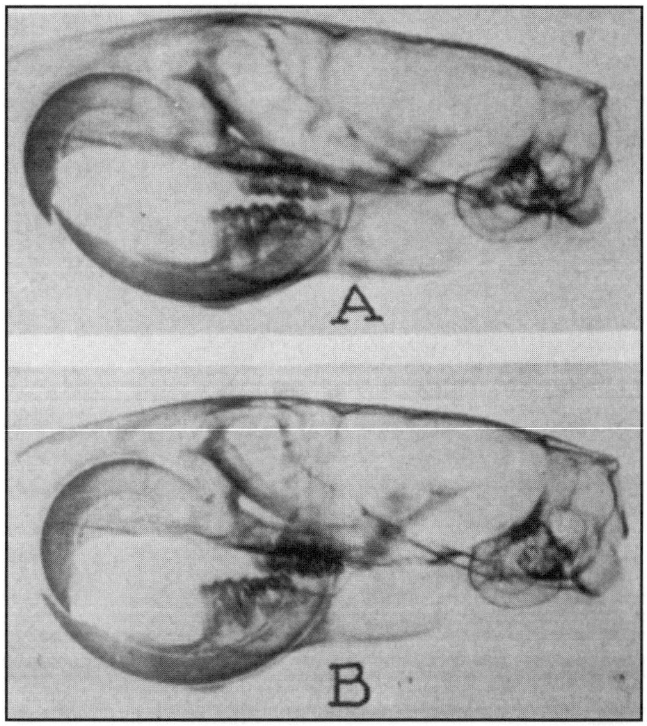

Fig. 6f. Sharpening rodent incisors by advancing the mandible.

structure reveals that they are composed largely of dentine which is covered by enamel on only the labial aspect and a very small portion of the medial and lateral sides. They constitute a pair of chisels by alternately passing each other when not functioning in prehension. The mandibular incisor passes its enamel edge up behind that of the upper on one stroke, thus sharpening the upper and on the next stroke it passes in front of the upper, thereby being sharpened itself. This type of movement requires a special joint, and this will be dealt with under an appropriate section (Fig. 6f).

7.

The Mechanics of Tooth Function: A Comparative Anatomical Analysis

Comparative Odontology

In order to understand how teeth operate, it is necessary to study not only the teeth themselves but also each of the factors that controls them.

The human dentition, the responsibility of the orthodontist, combines widely different functional patterns which are found in more specialized form in other species. Much of the confusion and controversy surrounding the dentition is the result of a limited awareness of the broad functional spectrum that exists in the various mammalian species and of the wide range that actually exists in the human dentition of different individuals.

The teeth are passive tools that function and react in response to the interplay of the tempomandibular joint, the bone of the mandible and maxilla, the muscles that move the mandible, and the periodontal ligament that holds them in the jaw. All of these have been modified or adapted to the unique characteristics and needs of each species. Our consideration must start therefore with the comparative anatomy of the design and structure of the teeth.

The Carnivorous Dentition

Probably the earliest highly developed denture is that leading to the Carnivora, the dental formula of which has been reduced to

Incisor	Canine	Premolar	Molar
I.3/3	C.1/1	P.M. 3/2	M. 1/1

The principles on which this carnivorous dentition operates are most apparent. The only teeth in these animals that are devoted to the preparation of food for swallowing are the so-called carnassials, which are the upper third premolar and the lower first molar. Their function is to cut flesh into pieces small enough to be swallowed.

The upper third premolars are tritubercular in design but markedly flattened in both crown and root in the buccolingual dimension. The middle cusp is the largest and highest, and the most posterior is next in size with its tip directed posteriorly. The anterior cusp is small and non-functional. The middle and posterior cusps present a marked, V-shaped interval between them which is the primary functioning part. The antagonist of this tooth is the mandibular first molar, similarly flattened buccolingually, with two cusps. The anterior cusp is only slightly higher than the posterior.

The Shear Principle

If one studies a pair of scissors, it is noted that when they are fully closed and viewed from above or below, only the tips of the two blades are in contact. As the scissors are opened this contact point moves back toward the joint as the blades progressively cross each other. Only one point on the edge of each blade can be in contact with a similar point on the opposite blade at any instant. This arrangement of a single, traveling point of contact is the most efficient cutting instrument known because it requires a minimum of energy to operate it. In the scissors it is made possible by the spring properties of steel, which are not found in living animals.

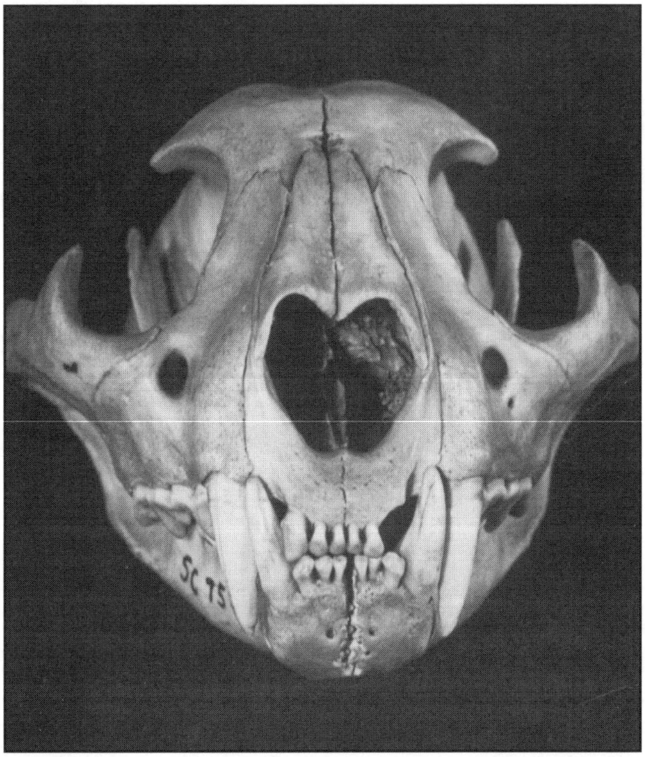

Fig. 7a.

There are, however, a number of ways in which the shear principle can be applied without this property of steel. The fundamental requirement for its operation rests upon the approximation of two blades at only one point. This can be met by two curved edges that are not congruent. Two convex edges facing each other or two straight edges moving in controlled arcs also could be made to function with a travelling point contact. All of these are found when one studies various types of teeth (Fig. 7a).

In the case of the carnassial teeth there are two slightly convex surfaces facing each other, the lingual of the upper and the buccal of the lower, but these surfaces are broken by the notch between the cusps. Hence, there are two sets of shears that face each other to trap and cut flesh. However, when the jaws are closed, the carnassial teeth of the mandible are completely lingual to those of the maxilla. Thus lateral mandibular movement is necessary, and this makes simultaneous contact of both pairs of shears impossible. In fact, if the jaw is opened slightly, there is no contact between the upper and lower teeth.

The temporomandibular joint of the carnivora is the most closely controlled of all animals. The condyles and fossa are arranged on a straight transverse axis, and there is no possibility of any anteroposterior movement. When the jaw is moved into function it shifts laterally until the teeth are in contact, and closure from this point is dictated mainly by the approximating tooth surfaces. Since these surfaces are curved, the mandible closes through two arcs, the closing hinge itself and the sliding movement in the medial direction.

But there still is another small arc to be reckoned with—albeit a very small one. The mandible of these animals is divided at the symphysis, with the two halves connected by a strong elastic membrane. The masseter and the pterygoid muscles attach to the inner and outer surface of the ramus at almost the same horizontal level so that their contraction tends to separate the mandible at its lower border. This imparts movement in the form of a slight rocking of each half and supplies a third arc of movement in the frontal plane. Through the integration of these three arcs, the functional side of the mandible is caused to move in such a manner that only one point of each shear can be in contact at any instant of time, and the teeth sharpen each other in the same manner as scissors or as one sharpens a carving knife.

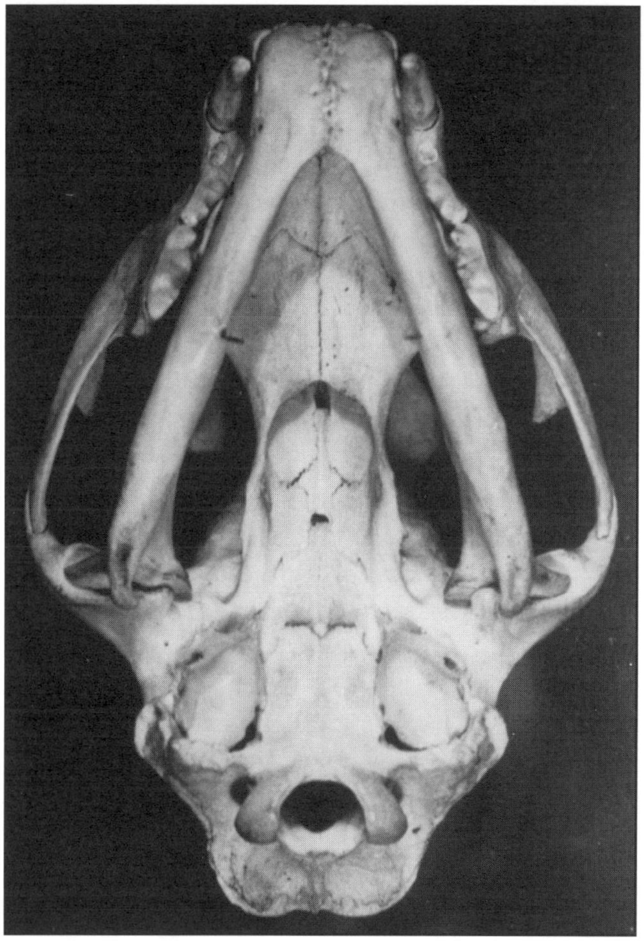

Fig. 7b.

The carnassial teeth are covered with very hard enamel that is extremely brittle. One can imagine what would happen to them if the jaw were to be shifted a little too far laterally and they were to come together end-on. They are prevented from doing this by the canine tooth, which finds its highest development in these animals. It is large, strong, and firmly anchored, the upper root extending almost as high as the orbit. In addition to being the killing weapons for the cats, they also play an important role as safety devices for the posterior cutting teeth. Being long, they prevent the jaw from overshifting and lead the mandibular tooth into precise contact with its antagonist. Considering the great horizontal force applied by the masseter muscle, it becomes apparent that these muscles in conjunction with the canine teeth have the same effect as the screw that holds the blades of a scissors tight together (Fig. 7b).

The great phylogenetic importance of the teeth

of these animals is further attested by the shape of the head, by the form of its individual bones, and by the specialization of muscles that control its jaws. The skull is short and flat, but width is imparted by the very strong and widely spread zygomatic arches. These arches give origin to the strong masseter muscles, whose function it is to maintain heavy lateral tensions on the teeth as the jaws are closed as well as providing anchorage for the usual crushing activity of the masseter.

The design of the mandible also deserves careful attention. The condyle lies at the *same level* as the functioning edges of the teeth, and behind it is a strong process which embraces the back of it. This postglenoid process in some species is so complete that the jaw can be disarticulated only with great difficulty even in the dried skull (Fig. 7c).

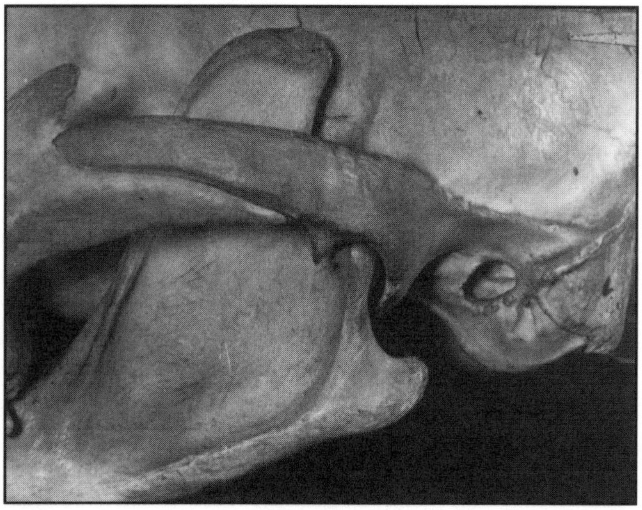

Fig. 7c.

The coronoid process extends upward to a much higher level than the condyle and even the zygoma. The powerful temporalis muscle embraces most of it and runs medialward and backward from it to envelop the entire top and side of the head. It must be remembered that this animal preys on living creatures and, if it were not for the design and extreme specialization of the joint and musculature, the jaw could be dislocated. The temporalis muscle holds the jaw firmly back against the postglenoid process and is closer to its specific function by its inherent responses. This is shown by the following experiment (Fig. 7d):

Shapiro denuded the temporalis and masseter muscles of freshly killed chimpanzees and opened the jaws sufficiently to place pieces of heavy card-

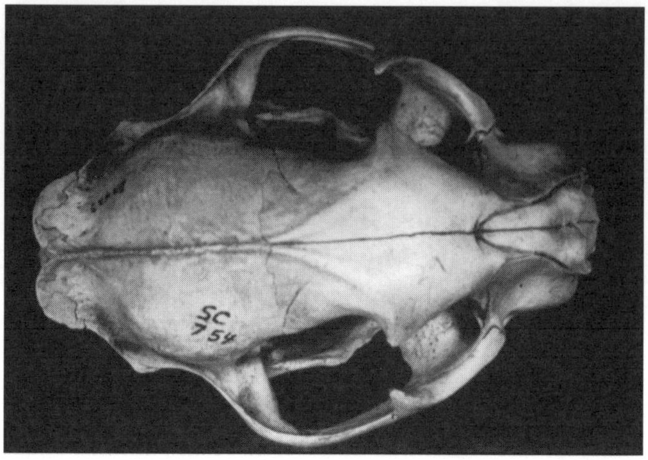

Fig. 7d.

board vertically between the upper and lower molar teeth. He then applied an electric stimulus to the masseter and the result was a slow powerful closure, such as would be employed in crushing hard food. When the same stimulus was employed to the temporalis, the jaw closed with a snap.

The Herbivorous Dentition

The horse provides a typical example of the herbivorous dentition. Although not a ruminant, the horse's dentition comes closer to the higher mammalian formula:

I.3/3, C.1/1, P.M.3/3, M.3/3

The canine erupts only in the stallion and even here is rudimentary.

We have already described the mode of formation of the teeth of these animals, so that it will suffice here to add that they may be thought of as tall, four-sided columns having a true occlusal surface, faintly convex interproximal surfaces, and grooved or fluted buccal and lingual surfaces. When they first erupt they have smooth occlusal surfaces, but this condition changes rapidly with wear so that they come to present a number of islands of dentin surrounded by low vertical walls of enamel, which makes them admirable milling surfaces (Fig. 7e).

The buccal teeth are arranged in series and constitute a separate unit on each side of the jaws, separated from the incisal segment by large diastemas. Each unit works independently. The arrangement of the milling teeth is different in the two jaws, those of the upper being set in an arc and those of the lower in a straight line. Further than this the lower

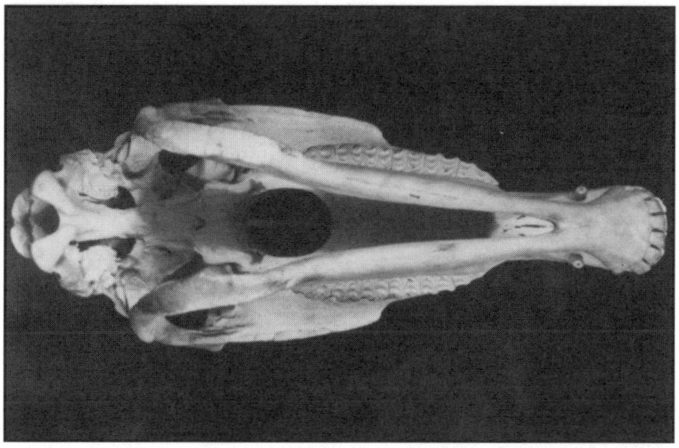

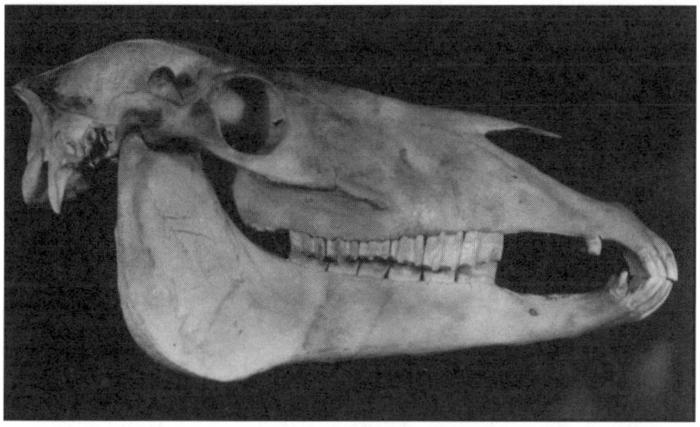

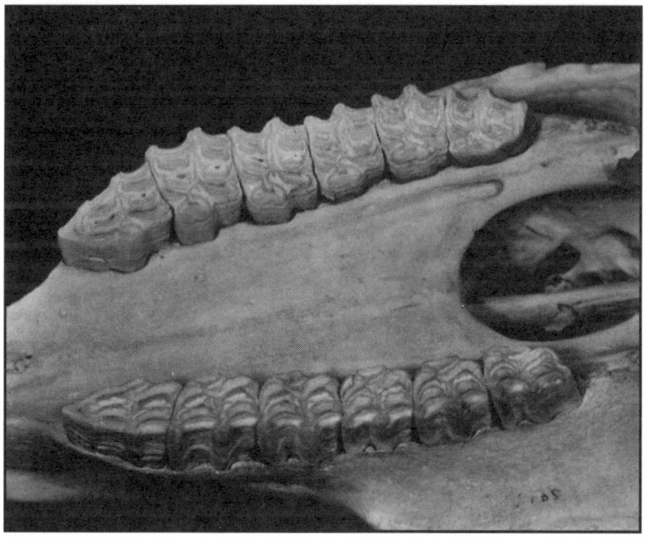

Fig. 7e.

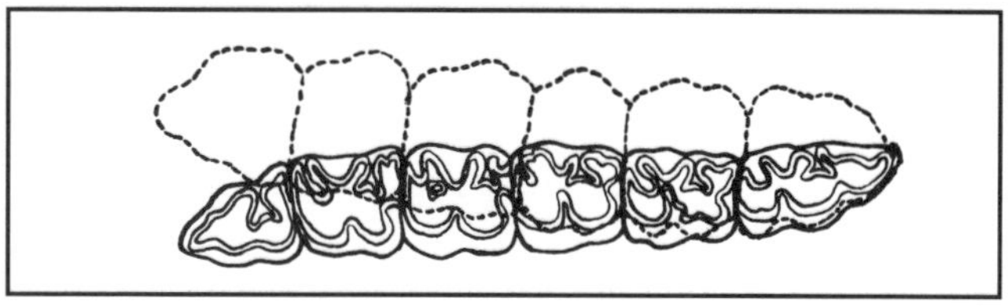

Fig. 7f. Diagram representing the occlusal relations of left buccal teeth at the beginning of the stroke. Solid lines represent the mandibular teeth; broken lines represent the maxillary teeth.

occlusal plane is quite flat anteroposteriorly, while that of the upper is curved with its concavity facing downward. Thus, when the jaws are closed in the centric relation, only the most posterior tooth in each segment appears to be in contact. From this point forward the teeth of the upper jaw are set further and further buccally until the most anterior is completely buccal to its antagonist. Since the occlusal curve is reversed, this finds this tooth hanging at a lower level than the occlusal plane of the lower so that the closed jaws are locked in the lateral direction (Fig. 7f). How then can this denture function in grinding?

When the temporomandibular joint is examined, it is seen that the condyle is set at an angle so that its axis runs anterolaterally posteromedially, and more importantly has a large "articular eminence" lying just anterior to it. Since the mandible is not separated at the symphysis, any movement of one side affects the opposite side. The condyle on the non-functioning side disarticulates the teeth of that side in the earliest stages of functional movement.

All of the above provisions in this dentition (and those of all grazing animals) also are designed to meet the law of the shear, with only one point in contact at any instant. If we consider the entire bucccal segment of teeth as though they were just two elongated teeth, an upper and a lower, the fact that they are different in shape, one straight and one curved in both the horizontal and vertical planes, it is immediately apparent that the requirement is fulfilled. When it is further realized that the mandible must work through three arcs: the vertical in opening and closing, the horizontal in swinging mediolaterally, and the frontal through the rocking that is caused by the articular eminence, one can realize the complex adaptation that has occurred. But even this is not all.

An examination of the occlusal surfaces reveals that these teeth wear in such a manner that the lingual sides of the lower teeth and the buccal sides of the upper are the highest. Thus, the transverse curvature is the reverse of that found in the unworn denture of humans. More than this, the occlusal surfaces of *both* upper and lower teeth are worn into concavities. Remembering the lesson learned from the rodent incisor, this tells us that the animal functions both during the lateral *and* medial excursions of the mandible.

An examination of the interproximal contact areas reveals clearly that the teeth work individually. When they first erupt, these surfaces are slightly convex and meet at only one point. With function, they are ground into each other in such a manner that they present faint "RSS" curvatures, which provide a small degree of lateral motion. When the first tooth meets its antagonist at the start of the stroke, it tends to push that tooth in the direction of movement and depress it. It is itself driven in the opposite direction and likewise depressed, while the adjacent teeth tend to remain stationary. As function passes to the next two teeth, the same thing happens to them and the first two return to their original positions. In this manner, considerable interproximal movement and wear takes place. The horse's denture is adjusted to wear and accident by the axial inclination of the teeth, which erupt continually throughout life. The posterior molars lean forward; the anterior molars lean backward. Interproximal wear is adjusted by the continual eruption of all the teeth, and they are kept efficient by the sharpening they receive through alternate medial and lateral motion.

In the various species of animals that live on grass or fibrous diet, one encounters all variations of the above arrangement of teeth. One common characteristic is their continuous eruption throughout life. Some present axial inclinations in the anterior direction, some in the posterior direction, and some are inclined in one direction in the maxilla and the opposite in the mandible. In all cases, however, the teeth converge toward each other as they approach the occlusal surface. In this manner function combined with continuous eruption tend to keep them moving together. In addition to these factors there appears to be a drift tendency in each of the species that is specific for that species. This tendency is especially marked in animals, like the elephant, where interproximal contact is absent and the molar teeth rotate down and anteriorly through the jaws throughout life, new ones erupting in back while old ones shed at the diastema in front.

In contrast to the head of the carnivorous animal, that of the herbiverous type is long, high, and narrow. These animals have many more teeth than does the carnivora, in addition to which there is always a large diastema separating the buccal from the incisor segment. The high, columnar teeth require jaws that also are high—to house them as well as to provide resistance against masticatory stresses which are predominantly in a vertical direction.

The muscles of mastication reflect their various degrees of importance by the development of the areas of attachment. The masseter is the most highly developed, since it is a crushing muscle. It takes its origin not only from the relatively small zygomatic arch but also from a strong masseteric ridge that runs well forward on the lateral surface of the maxilla. From here, the muscle runs downward to insert in a fossa that extends over much of the lateral surface of the mandibular ramus.

The pterygoid muscles also are highly developed and are oriented more like those in humans. The internal pterygoid attaches in a fossa on the internal surface of the ramus, similar to that of the masseter on the outer surface. The external pterygoid runs horizontally and provides the lateral swinging motion when it is contracted unilaterally.

The insignificance of the temporalis to herbivora is shown by the lack of development of the coronoid process and by the limited area of attachment on the cranium. These factors combine to limit the effectiveness of this muscle.

The Rodent Dentition

Although the rodent is the most widely distributed of animal forms, the characteristic specialization of the teeth, for which it is named, is restricted to the incisors (Fig. 7g). This enables the rodent to procure meals of many foods unobtainable by herbivorous, omniverous, or carnivorous species, but they provide him with no means of preparing the

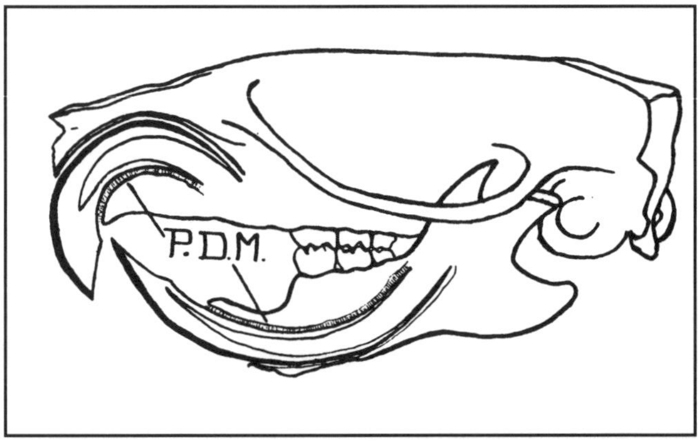

Fig. 7g.

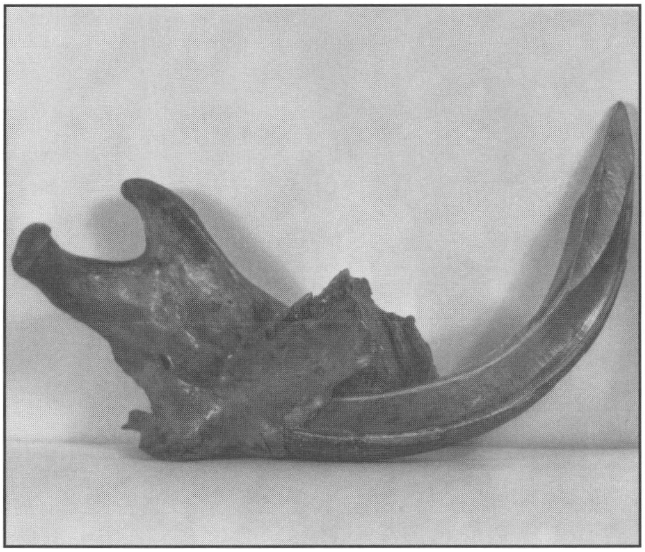

Fig. 7h.

food for digestion. This function is assumed by a segment of molars which is separated from the incisors by a diastema of relatively great size. The teeth of this segment reveal the nature of the diet to which the species has been adapted; they may exhibit the milling occlusal surface and the perpetual eruption of the grass and fiber eater (a rabbit and beaver), or the cusp/crown teeth of limited eruption that characterizes the omnivore (rat and hamster).

The extent of the diastema in the rodent, as well as the nature of the chewing movements of these animals, serves to emphasize a principle that they display more prominently than any other species. This is the inability to use the teeth of more than one segment at one time; one of the two buccal segments or the anterior segment alone. Further than this, the evidence presented by the wear patterns indicates that only a single point on a single tooth is in function at a single instant of time.

The mandible in these animals is divided at the midline, and the two incisors and sides can function independently. Shallow concavities are worn in the proximal surfaces of both teeth, indicating their alternate functioning. Alternate functioning is shown between upper and lower jaws even more strikingly in the lateral view of the head. The marked wear of only the lingual side of both the incisors keeps these teeth sharp.

The extent of the diastema in the rodents, as well as the design of the joint and the controlling musculature associated with it, exhibit adaptations not found in other mammals. As noted elsewhere the incisors, enamel-covered only on their labial surfaces, are kept sharp by an alternate passing of the lower tooth first behind and then in front of the upper.

The muscular control for these complicated movements of the two mandibles rests with a four-headed masseter, two of whose heads run forward from the angular process to the facial surface of the maxilla. These advance the mandible. Thus it will be realized that there are two joints, one for the incisal function and one for the masticatory. They cannot function simultaneously.

It also is evident that the two mandibles function alternately if one is to judge by the wear shown by larger species. Fig. 7h illustrates the medial view of the mandible of the giant beaver (Castorides Ohioensis). Despite the broken angular process, its form is that of a giant rat. Interproximal wear in this animal results in the two incisors becoming a point, and the shallow cavity near the end indicates alternate functioning of the two sides.

8.
The Eruption of Teeth

"While evidence on the mechanism of eruption is at present inconclusive and in the main tends only to negate present theories, certain conclusions may be drawn: (1) Eruption is independent of growth of the tooth itself. It is not dependent on elongation of root, growth of dentin or pulpal constriction, proliferation of Hertwig's epithelial sheath, growth of alveolar bones, or pull by periodontal fibers. (2) Eruption appears to be the resultant of a force acting upon the root of the tooth to extrude it into the oral cavity. Eruption is inhibited or deflected by mechanical obstructions (antagonist, deciduous predecessor, dense overlying bone, impactions) whose removal permits a full expression of the eruptive potential. (3) A significant correlation is suggested between vascularity of the periradicular tissue and the rate of eruption in both systemic (hypophysectomy, hypo- and hyperthyroidism, and local effects) vasomotor disturbances. Experimental modifications of the vascularity of the periodontal tissue may clarify further the mechanism of eruption."—Isaac Schour in *Experimental and Clinical Studies on the Eruption of Teeth.*

Even in the absence of proof pertaining to the exact factor or factors responsible for eruption, certain observations, investigative and clinical, have influenced this author toward the belief that the periodontal ligament is the agent responsible. To support this opinion the following evidence is submitted:

Carlson in 1942 studied the rate and amount of eruption of certain human teeth, using lateral cephalometric x-rays which were taken at six-month intervals over a ten-year period. The distances between the lower border of the mandible and the highest and lowest points on the lower central incisor, canine, first and second bicuspids, and first permanent molar were measured with correctional rulers (see Fig. 8a). Study of this figure shows that aside from expansion in growth the tooth crown remains at a constant level until root formation starts. With the beginning of root formation the distance between its open end and the mandibular border decreases slightly (2 to 4 millimeters), indicating a downward growth of the root into the subjacent bone. Following this slight downward growth of the root, all points on the teeth increase their distances to the lower border of the mandible. However, increase at the tip of the crown is greater than at the open end of the root, indicating that the tooth is erupting faster than growth of the root. This period of rapid eruption continues until the crown reaches the occlusal level, then slows and erupts only as the occlusal plane rises. After attaining this occlusal level, the roots are completed by growing down into the bone below.

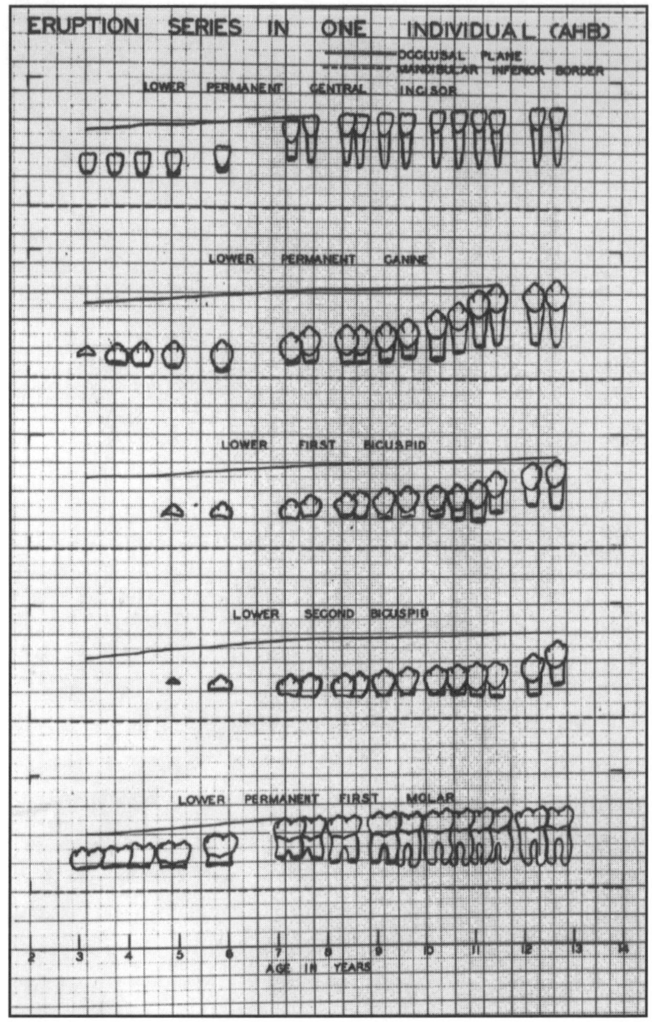

Fig. 8a.

The sudden slowing of eruption when the occlusal level has been reached should not be attributed to antagonistic forces such as the tongue or occlusion. The lower first permanent molar may reach its functional position months before its

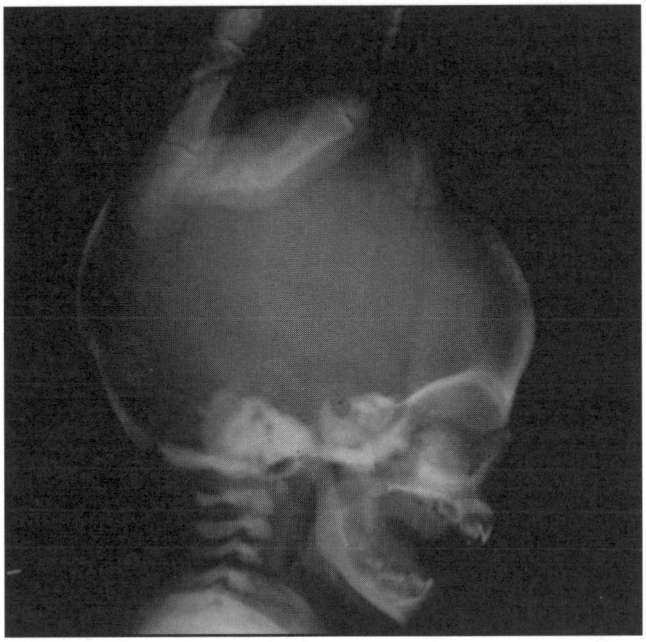

Fig. 8b.

antagonist appears, yet it does not erupt beyond the occlusal level of the second primary molar. In this, it resembles the behavior of other parts of the body which do not exceed their attained predestined size and form.

From the evidence cited above as well as from noting the eruption or orthodontic movement of pulpless teeth and teeth with arrested development of their roots, the author is strongly inclined to the view that the periodontal ligament is the direct active agent in the eruption of teeth.

A proper state of metabolism in the form of an adequate blood supply and endocrine balance must prevail to assure proper function of the ligaments, in the same way that fuel drives the engine which then turns the wheels. It is not the direct force supplied by the blood pushing the tooth into eruption, but it is some tension developed within or among fibers of the ligament raising the tooth into position. At present, the source of the tension is not known. There is no acceptable evidence that it is due to increased mitotic activity nor to rhythmic attachment and detachment of the fibers at either cemental or bony termini or in the intermediate plexus. It is quite possible microchemical examination of changes in the maturation and degradation within the collagen molecule itself may yield the answer to the source of the energy involved. Future investigations most likely will show several factors involved in the process of eruption.

The Placement of Primary and Permanent Teeth Prior to Eruption

The crowns of all the primary teeth have begun calcification at the time of birth and are placed in the jaws at levels indicating the order of their eruption (see Fig. 8b). The stage of their calcification is indicated by the neonatal ring which has been shown by Schour to be associated with the trauma of birth (see chart in *Atlas of the Mouth*).

In the deciduous dentition there is little difference in calcification or level of eruption between the upper and lower teeth. Beginning with the central incisors at approximately six months they are followed by the lateral incisors (9 months to 1 year), first molars (18 to 21 months), canines (2 to 2.5 years), and second molars (2.5 to 3 years). These figures represent means and standard deviations only and thus should not be used to judge normality or abnormality. Any large sample of children will reveal wide ranges of eruption, some having teeth at birth while others show none at one-and-one-half years. Extremes should merely alert the observer to the possibility of some untoward condition so that additional records or consultation may be anticipated. In cases of extreme precocity or retardation in the eruption of the permanent teeth, questioning the parent often elicits information that the same precocity or retardation occurred in the primary dentition. This should act as a deterrent to hasty orthodontic action: observation is called for.

There appears to be stability during the period of the complete primary dentition, but actually great changes are occurring throughout the jaws. The permanent tooth germs, an early development from the same follicles as their primary teeth, are left behind at their original levels during eruption of the deciduous teeth. Consequently, radiographs taken during the first three or four years of life show the incisal edges of the permanent central incisors at or above the root ends of the corresponding deciduous teeth. In viewing radiographs taken during this period, it must be remembered that the permanent teeth are lingual to the primary teeth (see Fig. 8c top and Fig. 8c bottom).

Associated with resorption and shedding of the primary teeth is loss of their supporting alveolar process. There are general misconceptions on this process as evidenced by some orthodontists advocating the clinical procedures of serial extraction,

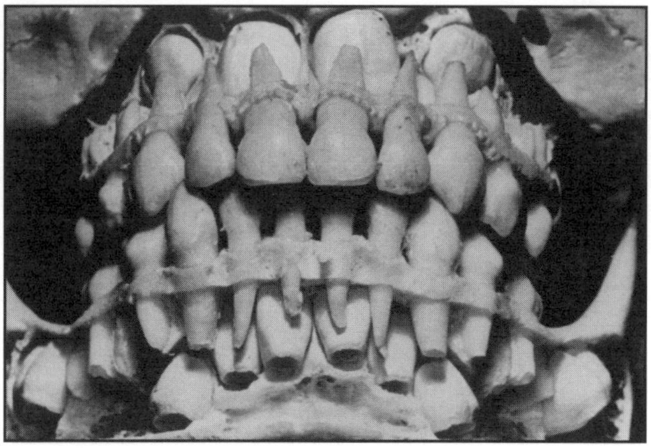

Fig. 8c top.

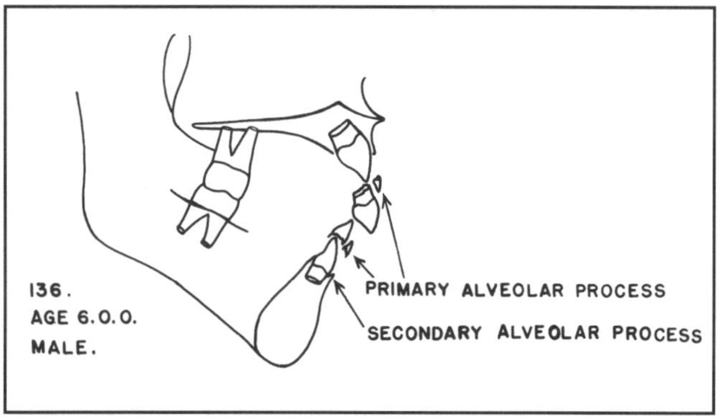

Fig. 8c bottom.

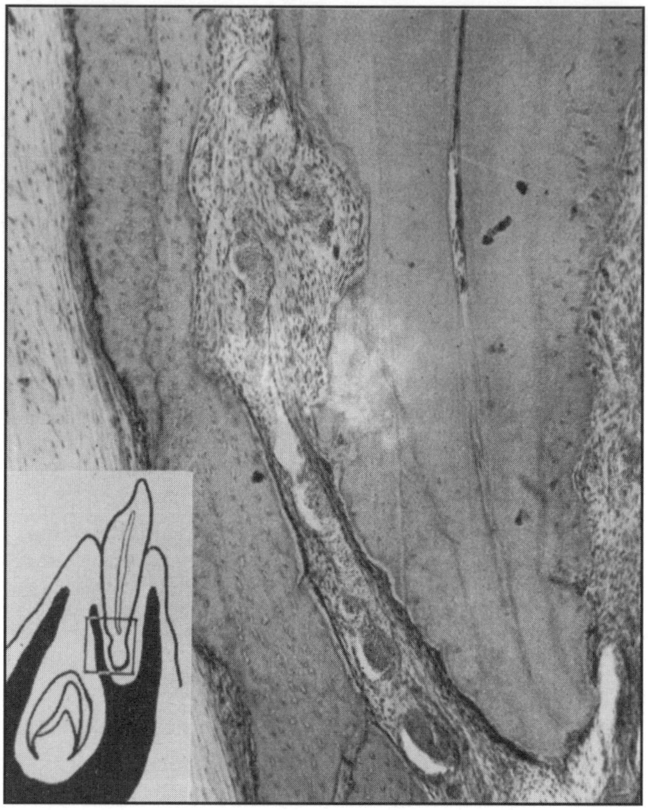

Fig. 8d.

the avowed purpose of which is to clear the way for the eruption of the permanent successors. However, 200 years ago Hunter pointed out that teeth do not erupt through holes already prepared for them; rather they remove the old alveolus and build a new process as they erupt.

The progress of root and alveolar resorption as determined from intraoral radiographs is misleading; both are judged by the degree of root shortening which is only part of the procedure. As in the building of the alveolar process, the periodontal tissues also are responsible for its destruction. Although radiographs show the first discernable resorption at the apex of the root, microscopic examination reveals it is not restricted to that area. Almost from the beginning alveolar resorption bays are found randomly scattered on both root surface and bony socket walls (see Fig. 8d). These areas are repaired and fibers reattached to them promptly so the tooth remains functional almost until it is shed—this in spite of a radiograph showing a funnel shaped absorption of the alveolar process tapering down to the neck of the succedaneous tooth. A similar condition is not infrequently seen, in intraoral radiographs of the bicuspid region. In these radiographs portions of the roots of the deciduous teeth are seen mesially and distally to the root of a fully formed and erupted bicuspid (Fig. 8e). Previous radiographs of the same areas show a larger than average bicuspid crown closely embraced by the tong-like roots of the deciduous molar. Extraction of the primary molar in such situations risks disturbance of the crown of the bicuspid, if not its entire removal.

It seems appropriate to state here that the resorptive processes mentioned above are not necessarily dependent on the presence of succedaneous teeth. Primary teeth without permanent replacements may be retained throughout life or may resorb at any time. Similarly, root resorption is found to occur in fully erupted permanent teeth. Such root resorption has frequently been attributed to orthodontic movement of teeth, with blame being placed on appliances that were too rigid, too loose,

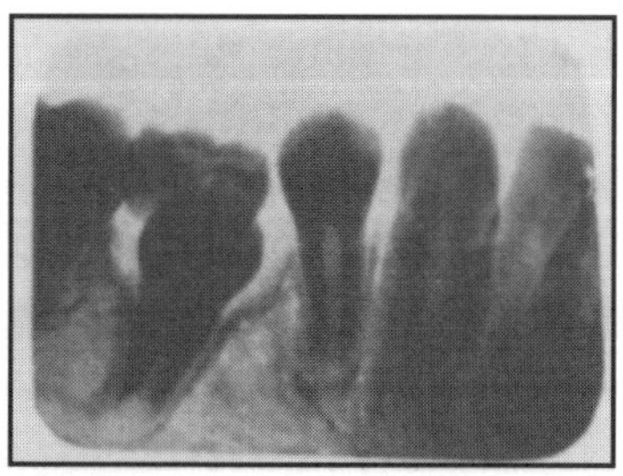

Fig. 8e.

continuous in action, or discontinuous in action. Becks found a greater than average incidence of resorption in subjects suffering from hyperparathyroidism. In short, little is known about the condition. If radiographs reveal resorption before orthodontic treatment is started, the patient should be warned that treatment may aggravate it but there is little danger of loss of teeth or their vitality. It should be remembered that fibers of the periodontal ligament in the gingival third or half of the root are responsible for the retention of the tooth. Considerable loss at the apical end of the tooth may occur without discernable effects except those seen in radiographs.

Eruption of Permanent Incisors and Canines

The primary incisors and canines usually erupt and assume their normal positions without crowding, but the permanent teeth which replace them are significantly larger. Serial radiographs taken from the second year of age onward reveal the course of events making possible the eruption and placement of the permanent teeth.

At the inception of the enamel organ the adult tooth germ is its full size, lying deep in the bone of the jaws which are large enough only to accommodate the primary dentition. Adjustment to the size difference is made by the arrangement of the permanent crowns. The central incisor edges lie lingual to the root ends of the teeth they will replace; being wider, they also extend behind the root of the primary lateral incisor. The permanent canine, the next tooth to begin calcification, is seen embedded beyond the root ends of the primary teeth in both maxilla and mandible. The incisal edges of the permanent lateral incisor are later located lingual to the permanent central incisor, being overlapped by both cuspid and central incisor (see Fig. 8f). How does this highly irregular arrangement result in the even alignment of the adult dental arch?

Since early dental writings there have been serious misconceptions concerning the manner in which the permanent teeth replace the primary teeth. John Hunter in 1783 wrote, "The jaw still increases in all points till 12 months after birth when the bodies of all six teeth are pretty well formed, but it never after increases in length between the symphysis and the sixth tooth; and from this time too, the alveolar process, which makes the arches of both jaws, never becomes a section of a larger circle, whence the lower part of a child's face is flatter or not so projecting forward as in the adult." From that pronouncement, the general opinion has been held that the permanent teeth are somehow fitted into the same bony arches which previously held the primary teeth, erupting through holes already prepared for them. This is

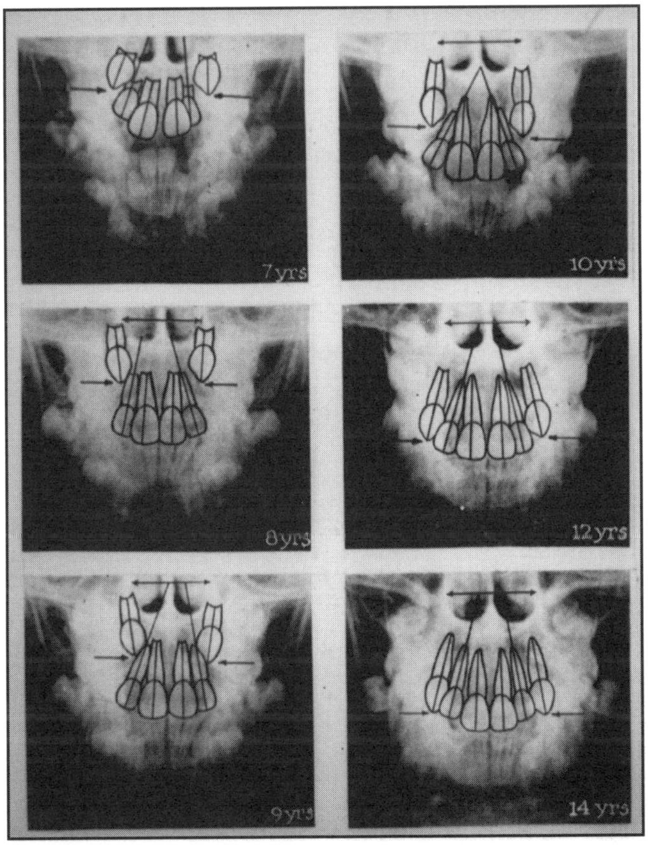

Fig. 8f.

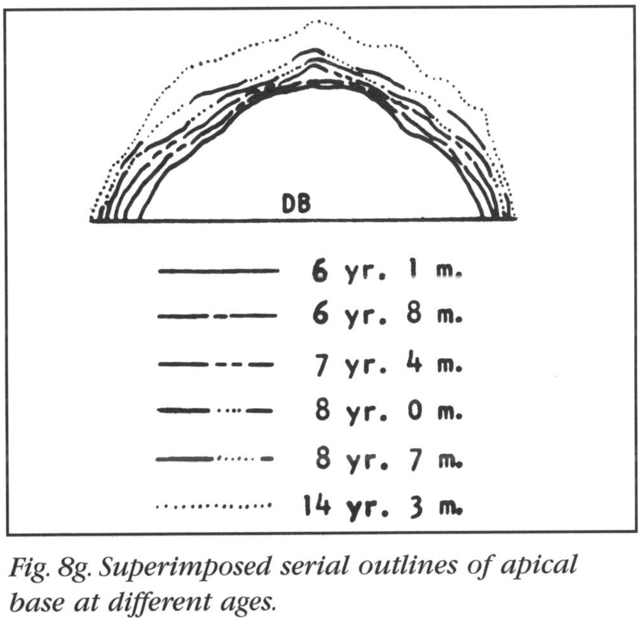

Fig. 8g. Superimposed serial outlines of apical base at different ages.

incorrect. As was indicated in the previous section, the alveolar bone of the primary dentition is lost with its teeth and new alveolar bone is rebuilt with the permanent teeth. This occurs tooth by tooth, escaping notice. But it would have been obvious if all the teeth had been lost at one time. As will be shown, the development of the alveolar arch follows the eruption of the permanent teeth in a downward and outward direction. Simultaneously, there is a continual expanded growth of the skeletal bone of the jaws (the apical bases), carrying the roots with it. As a result, the teeth are moved into a larger arc, becoming more upright as they are aligned (see Fig. 8g).

As all orthodontists are aware, the arrangement of the incisor and cuspid teeth prior to, during, and subsequent to their eruption is extremely variable. In some children some teeth are crowded, some are normally aligned, and some are spaced. Such diversity is due mainly to differences in the rate and timing of jaw growth related to the eruption of the teeth. If the rate of growth is low it could be late in relation to the eruption of teeth with consequent crowding. If, on the other hand, eruption of teeth is precocious the result will be the same even though growth of the jaws is proceeding a a normal rate. Teeth and jaws are derivatives of different body systems. Both are subject to variation and display considerable independence of each other. One difference contributes to their ultimate integration; that is, the manner of attaining adult size. The crowns of the teeth are formed as adult size while the jaws, dictating the position of the roots of the teeth,

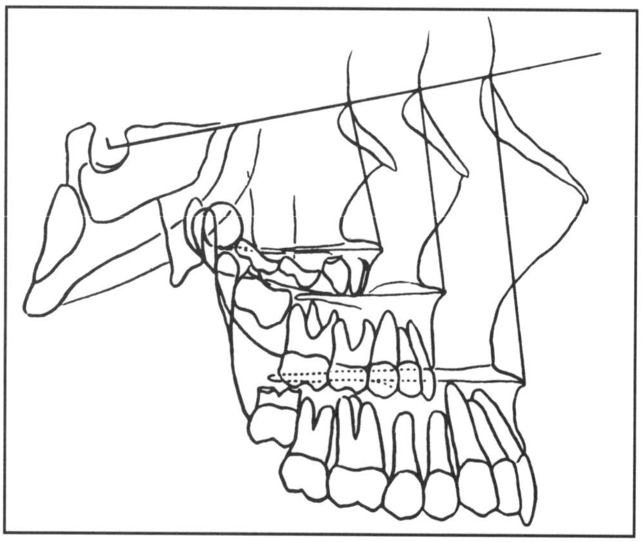

Fig. 8b.

grow continually from inception to adulthood. It seems apparent that crowded conditions during the growing years can only improve with time, particularly in Class I cases. Treatment prior to the attainment of sufficient growth is apt to prove disappointing.

An illustration (see Fig. 8h) portrays the progress of a child through this critical period. The gradual change in axial inclination of the incisors indicates that growth of skeletal bone at and above the root ends is slightly delayed in relation to eruption of the incisors and cuspids. Fig. 8i shows similar conditions in the mandibular arches of several individuals. The radiograph in the lower left corner portrays a condition formerly designated as "Ectopic Eruption," an obvious misnomer. With further eruption of the permanent lateral incisor both primary lateral and canine will probably be lost. Some radiographs show notches on the medial sides of the roots of the primary cuspids. These notches or resorption bays indicate the location of the erupting permanent lateral incisors before they were released by jaw growth. Radiographs from another child indicate that the permanent lateral incisors began their eruption directly below the deciduous canines and continued eruption during a period of rapid growth. Although they sheared the canine roots obliquely from apex to gingival line, the primary cuspids were not lost and the permanent laterals took their position in the arch.

Disturbances of Eruption

Failure of a tooth or teeth to erupt is a problem in differential diagnosis, since the failure may be

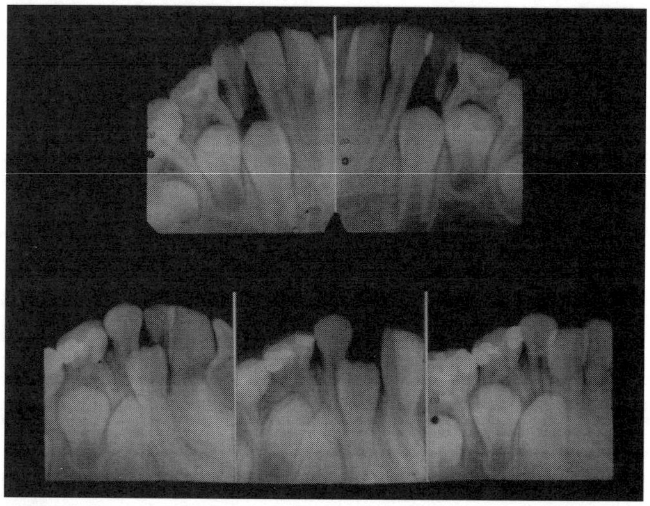

Fig. 8i.

associated with both systemic and local conditions. Systemic factors may include hypothyroidism and hypopituitarism.

In hypothyroidism, radiographs show the presence of teeth, but relative retardation of jaw growth is thought to be partly responsible for their arrested eruption. With early detection of hypothyroidism and the prompt institution of replacement therapy, patients with eruption symptoms can be restored to a nearly normal level. This was pointed out by Engle (1941) in his study of treated and untreated patients. This indicates that the symptoms do not appear until the offspring is independent of the supply of maternal thyroid secretion.

Hypopituitarism, anterior pituitary insufficiency, reveals itself by a lack of growth including that of the jaws. Although maturation of the teeth is delayed they ultimately attain normal size and form—but the jaws do not and crowding results. Replacement therapy in the human does not yield a large response.

Local factors which may be involved in delay or failure of eruption include impactions, a supernumary tooth in the path of eruption, tough connective tissue or bone overlying the erupting tooth, and ankylosis of the deciduous predecessor or even of its own root. In addition to these easily detected causes, normal eruption of a tooth may be disturbed by its following an atypical path of eruption. The mandibular third molar, usually, and the maxillary canine, frequently, execute extensive rotary and axial movements in order to take their ideal positions in the dental arch. Any arrest or delay of these rotations can result in impaction of the molar against the tooth in front of it or the entrapment of the canine in the bone of the palate.

Radiographs will frequently show the permanent upper canine lying in the bone of the palate. It was formerly a practice to uncover the crowns of such teeth, embed an eyelet in a hole drilled into the enamel, and attach a ligature wire. The canine was then drawn to a position where it could be banded. Recently, it has been found that the teeth will usually erupt spontaneously following removal of bone overlying the crown. Even unoperated upon they will sometimes go through extreme positional changes to reach their final location. Fig. 8j is an illustration of such a case and reveals the advantage to be gained from periodic records.

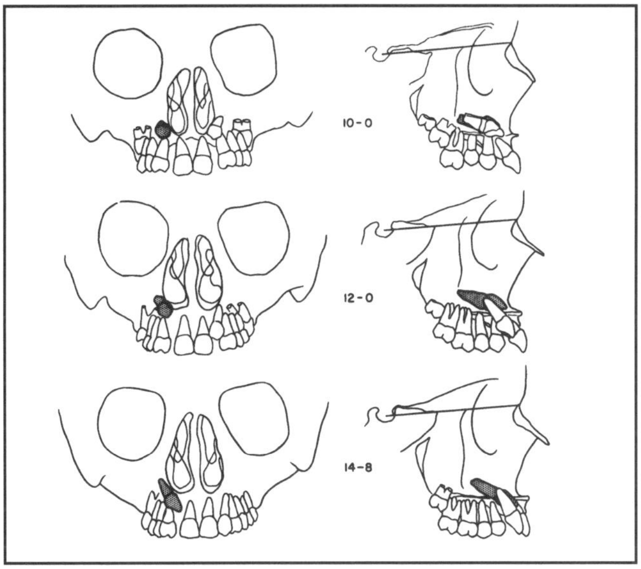

Fig. 8j.

A study of the gubernaculum in the dentition of the pig by Corollo et al. (1971) showed that removal of the gubernaculum or occluding its canal was followed by a filling in of cancellous bone and by a retardation and alteration in the path of eruption of the permanent tooth.

A more tenable explanation for the relatively high incidence of disturbances in eruption may lie in the differences between the variables of jaw growth and the variables of eruption. Jaw growth is a continuing variable proceeding in enlargement by imperceptible degrees, while eruption is a discontinuous variable involving the addition of fully grown units in the manner of cars being added to a train. It follows from this that only well-nigh perfect integration of the two sets of variables can result in uneventful eruption. If eruption is precocious or jaw growth lags there will be crowding at least of a temporary nature. It is at this point the orthodontist must exercise patience; time and growth are on his or her side, and careful observation over sufficient intervals of time usually will be rewarded.

Ankylosis or submerging of a tooth may occur during the course of eruption of any tooth and the associated development of its alveolus. It has been shown to be due to bridging of the periodontal space by bone, and however limited, the extent of the attachment eruption stops. In the earliest stages an ankylosed tooth can be identified by the hard bell-like sound emitted by striking it with a steel instrument. In contrast, there is a dull thud emitted by a tooth with a normal periodontium. In most cases a diagnosis can be made from radiographs which reveal absence of the periodontal space and discontinuity of the lamina dura at the site of attachment. More apparent is the submerging of the tooth below the occlusal level of its neighbors. All of these signs increase with time as more of the root surface becomes involved and appears to blend with the bone surrounding it. As the tooth continues to fall behind it may be completely enclosed. Ankylosis most frequently affects deciduous molars and first permanent molars.

The management of ankylosed teeth is fraught with risk. Any attempt to move them orthodontically will fail although they offer perfect anchorage for the movement of other teeth or fixed points of reference from which to measure certain aspects of growth. Ordinarily, the wisest procedure is to have them removed as soon as they are detected so that growth and eruption of other teeth may not be further delayed. Skill and care should be exercised and the operator should be fully aware of any peculiarities in the case. In the lower jaw, the tong-like relation of the roots of the deciduous second molar around the crown of the underlying second bicuspid can readily result in extraction of the permanent tooth with removal of the primary molar. In the upper jaw, the roots of the first permanent molar may extend considerably above the floor of the sinus and the site of ankylosis may be at the bifucation of the roots. Extraction of ankylosed molars in these circumstances may result in opening in the floor of the sinus.

Eruptive Behavior of Lower Molars

With the completion of the primary dentition, the relation between the teeth and the alveolar arch on the one hand and the mandible on the other begins to change. Until this time, the dental arch has seemed to be positioned directly above the lower border of the mandible and the anterior border of the ramus rises almost immediately behind the second primary molar—although more buccally than lingually. With the continual backward and divergent growth of the mandibular body, the posterior end of the alveolar process comes to lie more medially to it, a trend which continues until growth is completed. This divergence of the ascending ramus from the upper border of the mandibular body results in a triangular space behind the second primary molar, which gradually enlarges by resorption of the anterior border and deposition on the posterior border of the ramus. It is into this area that the permanent molars erupt in succession, but it should not be inferred that the relation of the ramus is the same as was that of the primary molar at an earlier stage. The eruption of each molar finds the ascending ramus further buccally with the result that the alveolar process appears to be an outgrowth of its medial surface. Intraoral x-rays of some individuals taken during and after the eruption of the third molar will reveal that tooth standing in a good axial inclination but with as much as the distal half of its crown apparently buried in the ramus. A glance into the mouth discloses it in full eruption with space between it and the ramus. (See Appendix II: Endnotes.)

Rotations Associated with Eruption

Seemingly all teeth exhibit rotary movements during their eruption. These are genetically dictated and species linked. In man, they are most unmistakably demonstrated by the permanent molars, particularly the lowers.

Seen only as a crypt in the lateral head x-ray of the newborn, the lower first permanent molar gives the impression of its forward, i.e. mesial, inclination and when its cusps begin their calcification the impression is confirmed. If a tracing of the cusp tips is made at that stage, a line connecting them can be taken to represent the occlusal surface and a perpendicular to the midpoint of the line can be taken to represent the long axis of the tooth. Successive stages treated in this manner will provide an accurate measure of axial changes in the sagittal plane

Longitudinal series of cephalometric x-rays from birth to adulthood reveal a gradual uprighting, i.e., distal rotation of the axis to take place until occlusion is attained, but the degree of change varies among individuals. In some the rotation is insufficient to prevent impaction against the root or neck of the primary molar. In the younger years, these will not infrequently free themselves with further mandibular growth. In other cases, the distal rotation may proceed too far, resulting in a distal inclination of the tooth. This does not seem to occur in the case of the first molar as often as in that of the second, but it may occur even in the eruption of

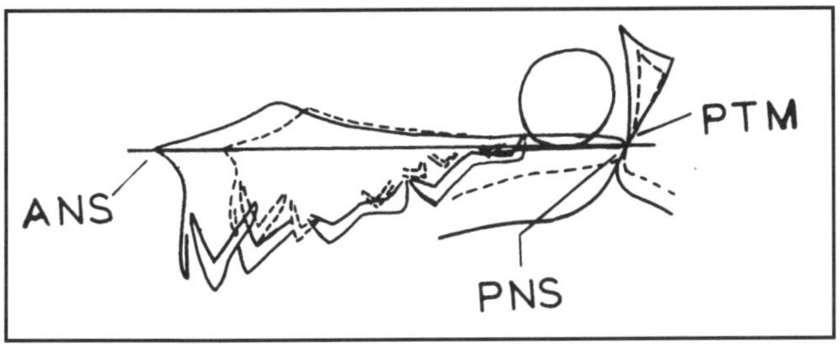

Fig. 8k.

the third. Occlusion with the upper teeth will usually improve the axial inclination of such teeth.

Rotations similar to those just described also occur in the transverse or frontal plane, i.e., buccolingually. Their study requires complementary posteroanterior cephalometric films. The earliest films of such series show the crypt of the first permanent molar almost completely buccal to the roots of the second primary molar which are, of course, well forward of it. When the cusps can be delineated the entire occlusal surface can be seen because of the mesial inclination of the tooth. Even at this stage, it also is apparent that it is also lingually inclined. Beginning with root formation and active eruption, the crown of the tooth is seen to move behind that of the second deciduous molar which lies ahead of it. Concomitantly, it rotates buccally to become more upright, but it does not attain a truly vertical position, its roots diverging buccally and its occlusal surface remaining canted slightly lingually.

The second and third molars erupt in a similar manner, but their rotary movements are progressively greater. Each completes its crown formation on a line connecting the inner and outer angles of the mandible, appearing to lie half in the body and half in the ramus in the lateral x-ray. In the frontal x-ray, however, they are seen to be completely lateral to the teeth already in the mouth. The second molar has a greater lingual inclination than that shown by the first at the corresponding stage, and this is even greater in the third molar. In some individuals, the inclination is so great that the occlusal surface faces directly lingual; that is, the axis of the tooth lies horizontally. Thus, when these teeth begin root formation and enter active eruption, their axes must simultaneously rotate buccally. Failure to attain sufficient uprightness results in their being caught in lingual occlusion. At this early stage their buccal rotation can usually be completed with the pressure of a fingerspring. Over-rotation, on the other hand, may lead to a buccal position, but this is more rare. Its correction requires a continuous force such as a criss-cross elastic operating in an upward lingual and backward direction.

Eruptive Rotations of Upper Permanent Molars

All tooth crowns complete their development within the *skeletal* bone of the jaws, and as they form roots and erupt they give rise to the alveolar bone that will hold them. In the mandible, the relation between the alveolar process and the skeletal body changes quite dramatically, particularly in the molar region while this is transpiring. In the upper jaw such changes do not occur, the teeth and alveolar process maintaining relatively stable relationships throughout growth. In this jaw rotary movements seem to be necessitated by the demand of the tooth germ for sufficient room to complete crown development before jaw development is sufficient to accommodate it in its functional position.

When first discernable in the lateral cephalometric x-ray of the newborn, the placement of the teeth was as follows. The deciduous tooth crowns in the maxilla all were found to be calcifying at birth and were arranged in a line with the central incisor closest to the free margin of the alveolar process, i.e., closest to the position of eruption. The lateral incisor canine and first and second deciduous molars each were a little higher than the tooth in front so that the last named was completely above the level of the nasal floor. The crypt of the first permanent molar in the lateral x-ray is seen to be the shape of a flattened oval vertically disposed and lying at or above the level of the apices of the roots of the second primary molar (Fig. 8k). It is closely adjacent to the sphenopalatine fossa, and dissections have shown that the surface of the maxilla in this area is sometimes deficient. It will be recalled that the posterior surface of the maxilla, like the posterior border of the mandible, is the site of the greatest anteroposterior growth of the jaws and accompanies their continual forward positioning. The teeth move with them, leaving a constantly increasing space between the distal surfaces of the second primary molar and the pterygomaxillary fissure. It is into this space that the permanent upper molars will erupt.

When the tips of the cusps of the upper permanent first molar are sufficiently calcified to be seen, they will not infrequently reveal the occlusal surface facing more distally than downward. With additional growth of the area behind the deciduous tooth, rotation of the permanent crown begins. As root formation and active eruption start, the tooth is seen to swing downward and forward towards its correct position. It frequently comes into contact with its antagonist while still tipped distally but with additional growth and rotation it settles into its full occlusion. Occasionally, it swings too far forward before reaching the occlusal level and impacts against the root of the primary tooth-root, causing resorption. Because it is still quite deep in the jaw it is not often that it can be freed by separation, and the extraction of the primary molar is necessary. Serial cephalometric films taken during the above described states and superposed on N-S and S registered will give the impression that the molar is dropping straight downward, but this is not the case. It is being carried forward as well by the growth of the maxilla.

The illusion is created by the fact that the rotation of the crown gradually brings the large mesiodistal dimension into the contact line of the arch from its original, almost vertical disposition. Once the tooth has reached its occlusal position it becomes apparent that it travels downward and forward on the Y axis. As with the mandibular molars, there may be pronounced rotation of the upper molars in the transverse or frontal plane. The degree of such movement seems to be correlated with the degree of growth that is attained by the maxilla during the eruption process. Hence, deviation from the usual course of eruption increases with each succeeding molar.

In cases where growth of the upper retromolar area has not provided sufficient space for its reception, the erupting molar will break through the tissue behind and above the tooth ahead, its occlusal surface facing buccally and distally. In the absence of occlusal interference, such teeth will be found to rotate downward and lingually with additional growth. Failing this, they must be brought into their correct bucco-lingual position with flngersprings or criss-cross elastics.

The ultimate results of the behavior of the teeth during their eruption reflects accurately the nature of the factors that operate to carry them to their

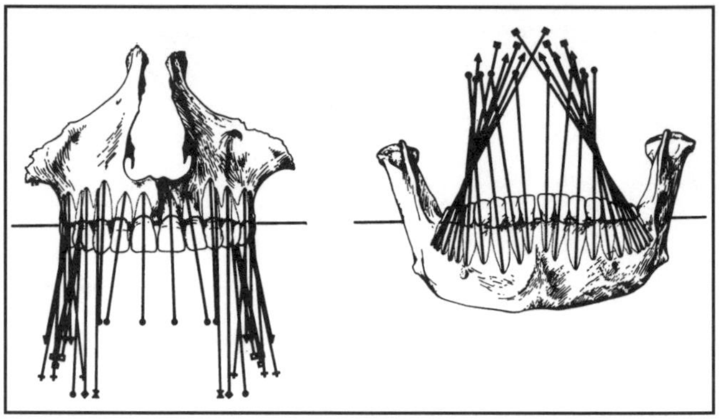

Fig. 8l.

final functional positions. Since all have their origins deep within the skeletal bone of the jaws, the outer form of the jaws and the relations between the jaws determine to a large extent the location of the apices of the roots after these are formed. The roots, with only a thin layer of bone covering their buccal surfaces, follow the outer surfaces of the maxilla and mandible. This is shown in collections of skulls where it will be seen that the ends of the upper canines and of the mesiobuccal roots of the first molars are frequently exposed. The same relation of the roots to the outer surface is equally true in the mandible but is masked in the molar region by an overlying external oblique line. Beginning

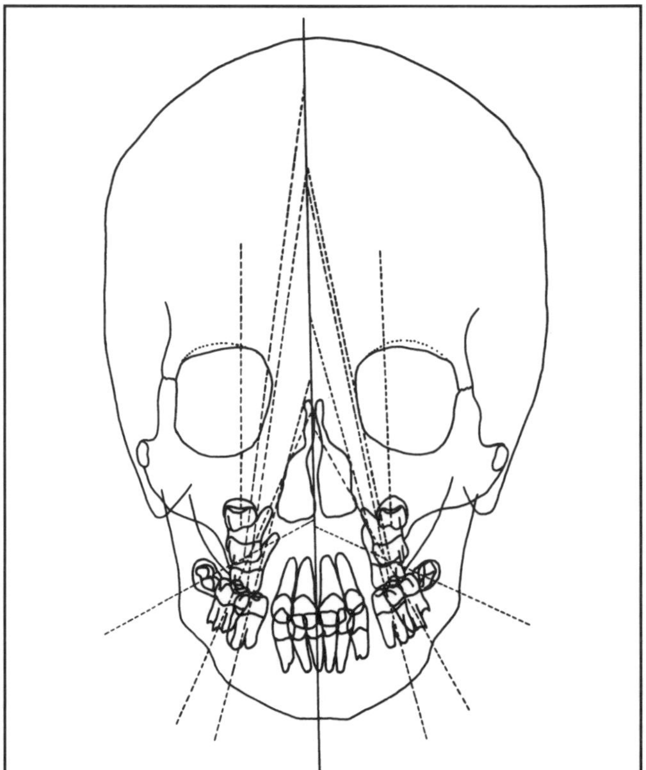

Fig. 8m.

opposite the first molar, this becomes a heavy ridge which ascends to form the anterior border of the coronoid process. Below the oblique line and ramus the lower border of the mandible diminishes in thickness to its smallest dimension as it approaches the angle.

Further evidence in support of the ideas expressed above is the study reported by Dempster, Adams, and Duddles (Fig. 81). Those workers located the long axis of each tooth in the 13 skulls having a full compliment of teeth in normal occlusion. These were enlarged by drilling to a size sufficient to receive a stiff wire. The drilling was continued through to the outer surface of the bone, wires were inserted in the holes, and various observations were made and photographs taken.

Fig. 81 illustrates clearly the differences between the arrangement of the roots of the teeth and the maxilla and those in the mandible. In the first, the axes are almost vertical when viewed from in front, whereas those in the mandible diverge progressively outward as the end of the arch is approached. Indeed, all of the wires from the buccal teeth emerge from the lower border of the mandible.

Reading list:

Broadbent, B.H. "Ontogenetic Development of Occlusion." *Angle Orthodontist,* 11: 223-241, 1941.

Carlson, Harry. *Studies on the rate and amount of eruption of certain human teeth.* Thesis (MS in orthodontia), University of Illinois, 1942.

Dempster, W.T., Adams, W.J., Duddles, R.A. "Arrangement in the jaws of the roots of the teeth." *Journal of the American Dental Association.* 67: 779, 1963.

Mason, Jack. *Behavior of the axes of human molar teeth during growth and eruption.* Thesis (MS in orthodontia), University of Illinois, 1957.

Ortiz Paiz, Manuel H., and Brodie, Allan G. "On the Growth of the Human Head from Birth to the Third Month of Life." *Anat. Rev.,* 103, March 1949.

Williams, Benjamin H. "Diagnosis and Prevention of Maxillary Cuspid Impaction," *Angle Orthodontist,* 51: 30-40, 1981.

9.
Studies on the Growth Pattern of Teeth

Teeth are ideal structures for the study of incremental growth, because they carry their growth or appositional patterns without change throughout life, in the same manner as a tree carries its seasonal rings. Many investigators have described the incremental lines in teeth, but it remained for Schour to employ them in a strictly quantitative manner and to lay down fundamental principles of this type of growth.

Schour's initial impetus was derived from the observation that injection of the salts of fluorine, particularly sodium fluoride, into living animals invariably resulted in a distinct line in the enamel and dentin of growing teeth. He quickly realized that multiple injections timed at specific intervals would yield information on the amount of dental tissue laid down during the period between the injections. Since sodium fluoride was known to be highly toxic and might therefore introduce metabolic disturbances and artifacts, Schour sought an innocuous substitute. This was found in alizarine Red S, the same dye employed in research on bone growth. The material gave an easily distinguishable, brilliant crimson line.

The early work was conducted on the incisor of the white rat. Since this tooth grows continuously throughout life, it was possible to obtain lines from the earliest deposit of material at the basal end of the tooth through complete formation at the erupted end. Much of this early work was done on adult animals, so few lines appeared in the molar teeth. The study of these lines in molars and incisors yielded important findings about the behavior of all of the involved cells.

All teeth start from the approximation of epithelial and mesenchymal tissues, assuming the form of a cone. The line of approximation becomes the dentoenamel junction, so dentin is deposited on the inner surface of the cone by odontoblasts while enamel is deposited on the outer surface by ameloblasts.

It had been quite generally assumed that the deposition of enamel and dentin occurred in even and equal layers and that the tooth represented the arc of a circle having a single center. Steadman in 1935

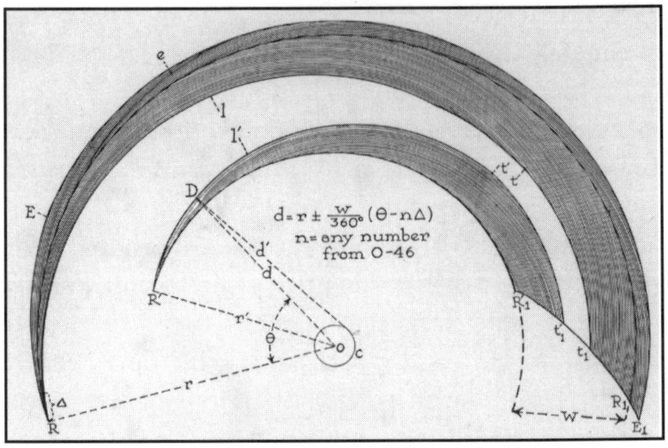

Fig. 9a. Diagram showing geometric construction of rat incisor, with formula.

(see reading list) disproved this by demonstrating that the form of the rodent incisor resulted from the operation of growth gradients, which yielded an Archimedean spiral (Fig. 9a).

In rodents the enamel organ does not completely enclose the cone, being deficient on those surfaces that will face lingually and on much of those facing mesially and distally. Both odontoblasts and ameloblasts grow away from the dentoenamel junction, the first growing in upon itself to become the pulp chamber and the second growing outward to ultimately become Nasmyth's membrane. The walls of the pulpal cavity in the rat become parallel opposite the crest of the alveolar process, indicating that no dentin is being formed beyond that point.

Having previously demonstrated the rate at which this tooth erupted, Schour was able to determine the length of time over which injections would have to be given in order to cover the entire span of dentin deposition. The greatest thickness of dentin occurs from the point where the pulpal walls become parallel to the cutting edge. Measuring this thickness and dividing it by the number of days over which injections had been given provided the average daily deposition of dentin. Although found to be 16 micra in the upper tooth, this was not all.

It had been demonstrated previously that each dentinal tubule was the work of a single odontoblast, and each enamel rod the work of a single ameloblast. Thus, the greatest thickness of the dentin and of the enamel represented the maximum work done by each of the two cells, and since it required an average of 40 days for them to reach their greatest thickness, it followed that the active lifespan of the dental cells of the rat incisor was approximately 40 days. This idea of a predetermined lifespan for a cell fitted into other growth investigations and explained other phenomena which, until then, had been obscure.

Schour and his collaborators next turned their attention toward teeth of more complex form: the rat molar. On the basis of what they had already established they were able to show:

I. That all the cells of a given tooth did not start to lay down enamel and dentin at the same time, but rather that each cusp had a primary center from which growth spread toward the periphery. This came to be known as the *locus gradient.*

II. That the various cusps appeared in sequence, not simultaneously, and that the teeth themselves did not all start at the same time. The order of appearance of the various growth centers was called the *time gradient.* The growth center always is found at the point where the most dental tissue will be formed—at the site of the tooth cusp.

III. Vital staining of incremental lines showed very clearly that such lines did not run parallel to the dentoenamel junction. Since the line laid down by the dye represented the tissue formed at the time of injection, this lack of parallelism clearly indicated that the amount of deposition per unit of time was not alike for all cells. The point at which the line was farthest from the dentoenamel junction represents the area where the rate of formation was highest. As indicated before, this was the cusp-tip region. Hence, the cells in this area are working at a higher rate than others, with the rate diminishing as the periphery is approached. This decline of the rate from growth center outward is called the *rate gradient.*

IV. Successive injections made at identical intervals of time revealed that the distance between the lines at any selected locus were not identical. The first two lines were farther apart than were the third and fourth, and so on. This was interpreted as indicating that the cell started its life activity at its highest rate and gradually diminished as it grew older. This was called the *age gradient,* since it seemed to be a phenomenon associated with the advancing age of the cell. When all of these observations are analyzed, one begins to grasp the concept that the difference between the original pattern or blueprint (dentoenamel line) and the final intricate form of the tooth rests entirely in the differences in the time of appearance and the operation of the above gradients of growth.

Although the same gradients probably operate in the determination of the form of bones, they cannot be clearly demonstrated by vital stains. This is attributable to the differences between teeth and bones in the attainment of their mature forms and size. Whereas teeth grow to their adult crown size and form before they erupt into function, bone must increase in size and strength as the body it will support grows. This demands constant alteration in its structure as it meets the increasing demands of growth. Only its proportions remain constant.

The precision attained in the studies on the growth gradients of the teeth pointed to the possibility that the onset of metabolic disturbances of even slight degree could be determined from teeth that were developing at the time.

Karnosh in 1926, Rushton in 1933, and Stein in 1936 (see reading list) had called attention to a contour line in the enamel which seemed to be associated with birth. In 1936, Schour recognized its etiology and called it the neonatal ring.

Because the rat incisor grows continuously throughout life, it offered opportunities for controlled studies on the effect of myriad constitutional and pathologic conditions on the calcification process in the animal body. These are beautifully described and illustrated by Schour and Massler in the chapter on teeth in *The Rat in Laboratory Investigations* (see reading list).

Reading list:

Karnash, L.J. *Arch. Dermat. and Syph.,* 13:25, 1926.

Rushton, M.A. *Dental Record,* 53:170, 1933.

Schour, I. "The neonatal line in the enamel and dentin of the human deciduous teeth and first permanent molar." *Journal of the American Dental Association,* 23: 1946-1955, 1936.

Schour, I., Hoffman, M.M., Sarnat, B.G., and Engel, M.B. "Vital staining of growing bones and teeth with alizarine Red S." *Journal of Dental Research,* 20: 411-418, 1941.

Schour, I., and Kronfeld, R. "Tooth ring analysis." *Archives of Pathology,* 26: 471-490, 1938.

Schour, I., and Massler, M. "Studies in tooth development; the growth pattern of the human teeth." Part I: *Journal of the American Dental Association,* 27: 1778-1793, 1940. Part II: *Journal of the American Dental Association,* 27: 1918-1931, 1940.

Schour, I., and Massler, M. *The Rat in Laboratory Investigation.* Chapter VI: "The Teeth." Philadelphia: J.B. Lippincott Co., 1942.

Steadman, S. "Geometric construction of the rat incisor," *Journal of Dental Research,* 15: 222-223, 1935.

Stein, G. *Ztschr. of Stomatol.*, 34:843, 1936.

10.
Musculature: Introduction

The usual method of teaching musculature on a muscle-by-muscle and group-by-group basis tends to obscure several important considerations of the system. Individually, each muscle would seem to have a single action dictated by its shortening between origin and insertion, but it has been demonstrated that adaptations have resulted in modifications in musculature that are reminiscent of those of the skeletal system where a single bone has come to serve a number of different functions. Different parts of a muscle may exhibit a range of function considerably beyond that generally assumed from the main direction of the fibers.

Muscles do not always act as might be expected from their locations and attachments alone. Although a single muscle may be the principal activator, it is only a part of the entire action picture. It is bound by fascial tissue to other muscles and to such structures as cartilage and bone, which not only serve as links of a chain but also modify or alter its direction of action. Great saving of structural mass as well as energy results from muscles acting in unison even though they may be widely separated and seemingly unrelated in function. Electric potentials can be demonstrated in the lower quadrant of the back of one side during mastication on the other side.

The mass of bone tissue can be held to a minimum by reinforcement and support from fibrous tissue acting to resist muscle pulls too strong for the bone alone to withstand. This is beautifully illustrated by the zygomatic arch, which can withstand the pull of the powerful masseter muscle when aided only by the temporal fascia and the galea aponeurotica running over the dome of the cranium. This was demonstrated by Eisenberg, who removed a band of temporal fascia one-inch wide along the length of the zygomatic arch of a Rhesus monkey. Twenty-four karat gold plate was burnished over the lateral and superior surfaces of the arch to prevent reattachment of the fascia. Biweekly injections of lead acetate during the six weeks before sacrifice provided microscopic markers to identify areas of bone formation. Post-mortem measurements revealed that the arch on the operated side was two millimeters (2 mm) lower and closer to the midline than on the unoperated side. Microscopic study revealed that active remodelling by resorption and apposition had changed it from the kidney-shaped cross-section to an elongated oval form. It was assumed that the unopposed contraction of the masseter muscle had induced these changes.

General Principles of Muscle Physiology

The discussion of anatomy and function will be more meaningful if we first consider some of the physiologic aspects of voluntary muscle tissue.

Although muscles were described as structures at a very early date, the phenomenon of their contraction and the source of their enormous power still is not completely understood. Their behavior has been studied at great length, however, and we can at least predict accurately what they will do under specified conditions. We must be constantly aware of these reactions if we are to deal with them effectively in the clinical situation.

Adjustment of Tension to Load

When resistance is encountered in the course of any muscular effort, the power of the muscle or muscles is unconsciously increased to overcome it. This is not a learned response. It is inherent in the muscle as shown by the following:

A spring from which weights are suspended will stretch an equal amount with each unit of weight that is added. If this same procedure is followed in the case of a muscle, it is found that the degree of extension lessens with each additional unit of weight until it will no longer yield. With addition of sufficient weight beyond this point the muscle will tear. Thus, it seems apparent that the adjustment of the muscle to the work to be done is on a basis of the number called into action.

Sources of Muscle Antagonism

Since muscles are constantly under tension, it follows that there must be one or more sources of outside force to apply such tension. There are two such sources. Muscles may be antagonized by (1) other muscles or (2) gravity.

In the case of muscle antagonism, there may be a condition where the muscles are equal and opposite in number, size, and location, as seen in the musculature of the back. The right side is a mirror image of the left when we consider the body bilaterally. Other conditions also may exist between antagonistic groups of muscles. Equilibrium may be established by a powerful muscle working against a weaker muscle or group of muscles, in which case the weak side is found to have greater mechanical advantage. In either case, all of the muscles are under a steady strain.

In some parts the tension is maintained on muscles by the force of gravity. This is particularly true in a dorsoventral direction, or, we may find a powerful group being antagonized by gravity plus the pull of weak muscles. Under any of the above conditions the net effects are equal and opposite and the antagonistic forces maintain a continuous state of equilibrium.

Reciprocal Innervation and Inhibition

When a muscle begins to contract (protagonist), it would seem that additional tensions would be set up in the opposing group (antagonists), which would inhibit, or at least limit, movement. This is not so. Sherrington demonstrated that there was a reflex arc set up between the stimulated muscle and its antagonists which inhibited the tension in the antagonists. Under this secondary impulse, the antagonists relax or stretch at a rate proportional to the contraction of the protagonist. The arc does not go through the brain, but only through the cord as shown by experiments with decerebrated cats. Some motion may even be induced by gravity by the inhibition of muscles which work against gravity.

Disturbance of the State of Inertia

Inertia is that property of matter which causes an object at rest to resist movement, or if in motion to resist arrest of that motion. In other words, more power is required to start motion than to maintain motion once it has started. This is just as true in the animal body as in the inanimate world.

Steindler of the University of Iowa conducted investigations on outstanding performers in many fields of sport and demonstrated that in every motion made there was preliminary activity of associated muscles which resulted in a disturbance of the state of inertia. One might say that this was a matter of throwing things out of balance. A good example is our need to fall forward before beginning to walk. After we have fallen a certain distance, we catch ourself with one foot. In this case, gravity is permitted to disturb the state of inertia by an inhibition of the back muscles. Through devices of this sort there is a great saving of energy.

The engineer employs gears of different sizes to start the motion of an automobile (overcome inertia) and to maintain it after it is in motion. The consumption of energy (gasoline) may be the same at both gear ratios, yet the speed of motion differs greatly. There is a great saving of energy when an automobile can enlist gravity by starting on a downgrade.

Other Functions of Skeletal Muscle

The voluntary musculature considered thus far must be thought of as serving the skeletal system primarily by providing for support of the body and the movement of its parts. Some of these muscles also act to stabilize the framework from which other muscle systems can perform nonpostural functions such as respiration and movements of the tongue, pharynx, and soft palate.

Chemistry of Muscle Contraction

Much work has been done on the chemistry of muscle contraction in an attempt to explain how it occurs. It was known fairly early that muscle tissue contained significant amounts of stored sugar in the form of glycogen, a known source of quick energy. It also was known that one of the chief products of glycogen breakdown was lactic acid, and that lactic acid always was present following muscle activity. The puzzling facts remained, however, that there seemed to be less lactic acid formed during muscular activity than would be expended from the amount of glycogen consumed, and also that even the amount of glycogen could not yield the amount of energy that was known to be liberated. Ultimately, it was discovered that there were intervening stages, and new techniques had to be developed that could "stop" the activity at these various stages. This was accomplished by quick freezing in liquid CO_2, after which the tissue was ground up and subjected to chemical analysis. This method led to the discovery of a number of intervening products and on the basis of these a logical chain of events was worked out.

There is present in resting muscle a small amount of hexosemonophosphate, which is markedly increased in activity. It is now generally believed that glycogen is first converted into a labile form of hexosephosphate and that this substance undergoes a series of changes which ultimately result in lactic acid. The greatest mystery was cleared up, however, when it was realized that this was not the end of the reaction. The formed lactic acid is next transformed into another series of substances through an oxidative process which ultimately resynthesizes it back into glycogen. There is thus a cycle of chemical reactions which uses all but a trace of the lactic acid and permits prolonged activity in relation to the amount of glycogen originally involved. Nevertheless, the trace of lactic acid that *is* left over and is constantly being added to during contraction, ultimately builds up to the place where it inhibits further action. We say the muscle is fatigued.

The All or None Law

A muscle is a bundle of very small individual muscles or fibers, each capable of acting independently. When such a fiber is stimulated it is found that any stimulus that will incite any response brings about complete or maximum contraction. We say the fiber responds "all or none."

Muscle Tonus

A muscle at complete rest is slightly shorter than one which has been freshly killed. This might imply either that a difference exists in the chemical tension in the living and dead states or that all of the fibers were partially contracted. However, a completely anesthetized muscle acts in the same manner—like a dead muscle.

If a freshly prepared muscle is tested by means of delicate galvanometric methods, it is found that no response is elicited from most of the fibers. Some fibers, however, do give a definite current. If the anode is held on such fibers for any length of time, this response dies away and now may be found in a fiber that was previously negative. It thus seems apparent that a few fibers of a resting muscle are completely contracted for short periods of time, thus giving tone to the entire muscle. (It must be realized that muscle fibers do not run the full length of the muscle but are interwoven with each other.) It is thought that after the contracted fibers have built up waste products, principally lactic acid, their threshold rises and stimulation can no longer bring about response. The stimulation then passes to another fiber and the previous worker relaxes and restores its glycogen. Thus tonus does not contradict the "all or none" law, but rather is the result of the total contraction of a few fibers acting on the entire muscle.

Resting Length of Muscle

The length of any muscle seems to be a genetic characteristic, but its physiology permits a certain degree of latitude in the direction of shortening. A muscle cannot be maintained beyond its genetic resting length. On the other hand, if the attachments of a muscle are closer together than the normal resting length of the muscle (as in undergrowth of bones or in accidents), the muscle shortens until the right amount of tonus is present. In such an instance more fibers are involved than would normally be the case.

It seems that muscle must act against a certain degree of tension and will shorten until this tension is established. This property of muscle has a significant bearing in the treatment of fractures of either bones or tendons. If, for instance, the tendon of Achilles is fractured and is not immediately refastened surgically, the gastrocnemius and soleus muscles shorten until the tendon is pulled well up the leg. In fractures of bones to which voluntary muscles are attached, the fragments involved will be pulled in the direction of the shortening muscle until the muscle meets sufficient resistance to stop the action.

11. Muscle Physiology of Head and Neck Region

Maintenance of Head Posture and Relationship of Parts

It was thoroughly established by Sherrington that the same motor impulse that caused one set of muscles to contract caused an inhibition of tonus in their antagonists. Thus, the rest position of any movable part may be taken as an equilibrium between all of the forces operating upon it. If these forces happen to be entirely muscular, there is an equal pull on both sides of the part through a state of tonus. Thus, even a rest position must be viewed as a dynamic condition.

There is no better place to examine or demonstrate this principle than in the upright posture of humans (Fig. 11a). One has no difficulty in visualizing muscular equilibrium when one views such a symmetrical arrangement as the two sides of the back. The problem is quite different, however, when the body is viewed from the side. In order to have the same static equilibrium here, it would be necessary that the line of gravity pass through the articulating surfaces on all of the joints supporting the body. Steindler has pointed out in his "Normal and Pathologic Locomotion of Man" that the center of gravity actually passes through few of the joints and that therefore there must be an antagonism to gravity set up by the powerful musculature of the back on the one hand, and the musculature plus the force of gravity in front. The truth of this contention is beautifully shown when a person faints while standing erect. The knees and ankles buckle and the body pitches forward. Steindler points out that for every movement of the body, there is a definite amount of inertia to be overcome, a definite amount of balance to be disturbed. In many parts, the body is so designed that the force of gravity initiates movement, as in walking. Here we permit ourselves to relax and start to fall forward, catching ourselves with one foot or the other. Walking, then, becomes a matter of alternating falling forward and placing the foot to stop the fall.

In the case of the head, there is an even more complicated system. Here we have what amounts to a globe set on top of a column of spools—hardly a stable arrangement. It is easy to see and understand the action of the postcervical muscles (semispinalis, trapezius, splenius, sternomastoid), and were there another similar group running from the front of the head, in the region of the forehead, to the thorax, we could readily understand the resulting balance. We know that we have the balance, but we have no such group of muscles. How, then, is the posture of the head maintained? In the head, the greater part of the weight lies anteriorly to the axis, the head falling forward when complete relaxation occurs. Thus, gravity does at least part of the work of balancing the head.

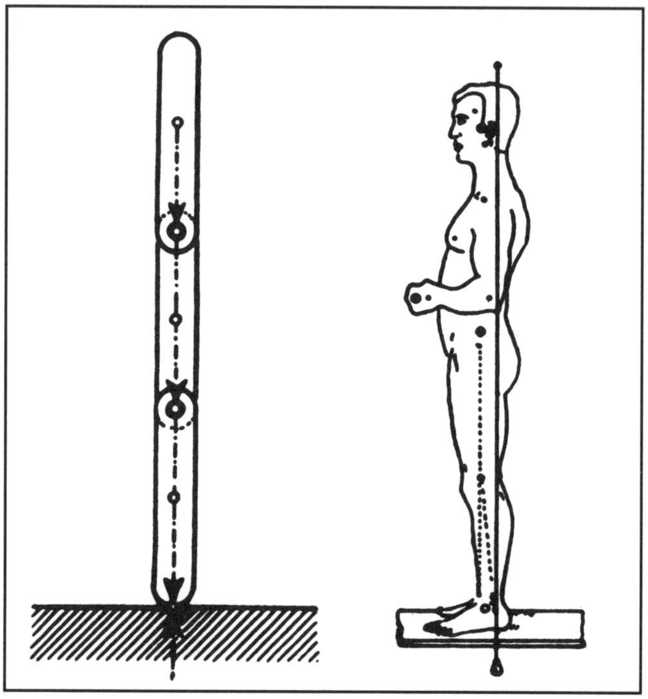

Fig. 11a.

When search is made for the more dynamic factors of resistance to the powerful postcervical group, it is found that a series of muscle groups act together. Each group has its own specific function or functions, but at least part of its work is this cooperative effort in behalf of posture maintenance. The superior group is the masticatory musculature (masseter, temporal, and internal pterygoid). Without exception, these muscles have their origin on the cranium and run to a movable bone, the mandible. Thus, they are capable of making a unit of cranium and jaw by clamping them together. A moment's reflection reveals, however, that even now they would not antagonize the posterior neck muscles. Without connection between mandible and thorax, the head would be tipped back. This connection is supplied by the suprahyoid and infrahyoid muscle groups, the first group (geniohyoid, mylohyoid, stylohyoid, and digastric) running from mandible and cranial base to the hyoid bone and the latter (sternothyroid, sternohyoid, and omohyoid) running from hyoid bone to thorax. Thus, we have three muscle groups that span the gap between cranium and operating base, or thorax, and control two movable bones. It is likewise apparent that the middle face, exclusive of the zygomatic arches, plays no part in the positioning of those movable bones.

Let us now imagine the head being held normally and motionless in the position of erect posture. Such a position is maintained by the antagonistic pull of the muscles on the back of the neck on one hand, and the force of gravity plus the three enumerated sets working together on the other hand. Suppose we disturb this balance by swallowing. In deglutition, it is necessary to elevate the hyoid bone, which means the contracting of the suprahyoid muscles. If this group is contracted, it would have just as strong a tendency to depress the mandible as to elevate the hyoid. seems obvious, therefore, that additional tension must be generated in the masticatory group to prevent the downward displacement of the mandible. The fact that this is true can be easily demonstrated by placing the fingers lightly on the temples and swallowing. Atthe instant of elevation of the hyoid, a pulse of contraction will be felt in the temporalis.

A similar phenomenon may be demonstrated in mastication. In spite of the rather extensive and violent movements of the mandible, the hyoid bone is relatively stable. Indeed, it is only in wide opening movements that the hyoid bone shifts to any extent. The excellent fluoroscopic moving picture, *Physiology of Mastication* by Klatsky, shows these points.

Thus, it is seen that the muscles lying anteriorly from the vertebral column, i.e., the masticatory, suprahyoid, and infrahyoid groups, have as their roles not only their own specific functions, but also a team play behind these which helps to maintain the posture of the head. This coordination permits mastication, deglutition, and speech without any accompanying nodding of the head.

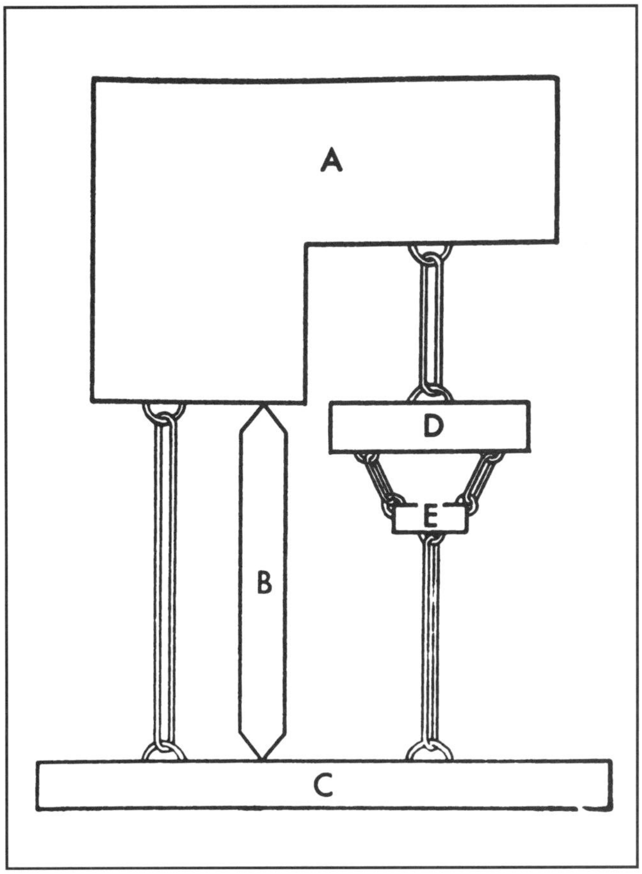

Fig. 11b. Diagrammatic representation of the equilibrium of the head skeleton.

The state of equilibrium in the human head is diagramed in Fig. 11b. The different skeletal units, designated A, B, C, and D, are represented by blocks connected to each other by elastic bands and held under tension by the prop, B, which is pointed at both ends to indicate its extreme instability. It scarcely needs mentioning that an increase in tension in any single elastic would require an increase in tension of all if the position of the blocks were to be maintained. Similarly, the elevation of D by the elastic above it would have to be accompanied by a corresponding slackening of the elastics below it if movement of A elsewhere is to be prevented.

The External Pterygoid Muscle

It will have been noted that the external pterygoid muscle, although one of the masticatory group, has not been included in our consideration of the muscles thus far. The reason for this lies in the fact that it does not contribute to the superoinferior position of the mandible, as do the other three. Actually, it lies more or less at right angles to the suspensory group and may be looked upon as a disturber of their equilibrium. On the other hand, it does play a major part in the anteroposterior positioning of the mandible.

Arising from the external pterygoid lamina and running horizontally backward and lateralward to the neck of the condyle, its tonus would tend to draw the mandible forward. It is antagonized by the horizontal fibers of the temporalis, which run forward to insert into the coronoid process. In the absence of modifying factors the equilibrium between these two muscles determines the anteroposterior position of the condyle.

Individuals who have suffered the loss of function of the external pterygoid through condylectomy or paralysis reveal the consequences in radiographs of their opening movements. At first, the opening movement is extremely limited, but as the hyoid musculature accommodates to the new functional demand, it responds as is illustrated in Fig. 11c. The mandible exhibits a rotary hinge-like motion as the hyoid bone is pulled to a constantly lower position to gain mechanical advantage. Only in the final extreme stage is any forward movement of the top of the ramus observed in this case, and this was due to the movement of the opposite side which was not operated upon. The extreme position of the hyoid bone precludes breathing at this time.

As additional evidence that the external pterygoid is the main source of power in mouth opening, it must be recalled that protagonists and antagonists which induce the opposite movements in actions such as opening and closing the mouth are supplied by the same motor nerve. The external pterygoid is one of the masticatory group that is supplied by the fifth nerve. The suprahyoids are innervated by the seventh and twelfth nerves. Also, when a sustained effort is made to open the mouth against resistance, fatigue occurs first in the region of the joint, not in the floor of the mouth. Thus, it seems that the contracting of the anterior suprahyoid muscles serves the function of insuring the stability of the hyoid bone in the interest of respiration, rather than the opening of the jaws.

In marked contrast to the arrangement in the human body is that found in four-footed animals. In these forms, the long head is carried in a horizontal

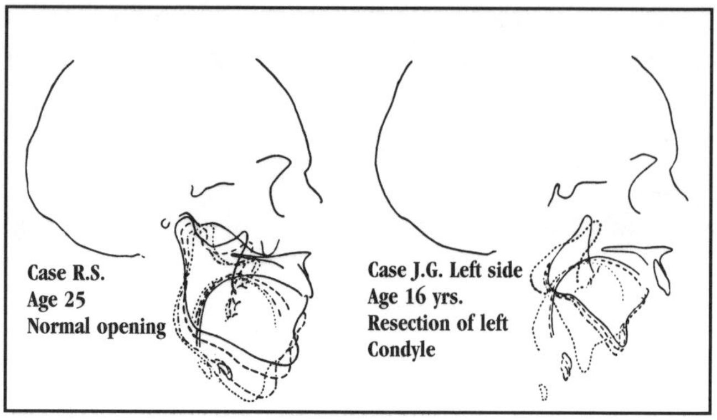

Fig. 11c.

position in an almost direct line with the spinal cord, the gut, and the respiratory intake. The constant tendency for the head to drop is resisted by powerful dorsal muscles which run well down the vertebral column and are given additional effectiveness by a heavy nuchal ridge and temporal muscles which cover the back of the cranial vault. There is little interdependence between the muscular control of head posture and mastication.

One of the best examples of muscular coordination can be seen in the opening movement of the mandible. Beginning from the resting position of the mandible, with all of the muscles in a state of equilibrium, the external pterygoid begins to contract. This would result in a straight forward movement of the mandible were it not for the slope of the articular eminence which deflects the bone downward. Any downward movement will lead to increased tension in the remaining three muscles of the masticatory group (masseter, internal pterygoid, and temporal), but such tendency is offset by reciprocal inhibition of those muscles. Simultaneously, the anterior suprahyoid group must exercise constantly increasing tension between the chin and the hyoid bone to prevent closing of the airway. This aids in the opening movement.

In 1906, Chissin published a paper in the German anatomic literature under the title "On the Opening Movement of the Mandible and the Part of the External Pterygoid in the Same." Apparently it was overlooked, even in Europe, because is does not appear in any bibliography until 1937. By very simple and direct means, Chissin demonstrated that the opening movement was not due to the simple lever action as generally assumed. The base from which he made his observations was a simple frame, equipped with ear rods and held in place with a large elastic band around the head. This frame had holes on the outside in line with the ear rods to receive plugs of a face bow, which thus could be rotated around the ear holes. The outer frame carried a block with a sliding scale which permitted measurements from its end to the ear hole. Initial points were located indicating the lower central incisor, the chin point, the angle of the mandible, and the center of the condyle with the teeth occluded. These points were connected with straight lines and a pattern was laid out and cut from cardboard to be used as a template. At four stages opening from occlusion to wide open, it was necessary to locate only the incisal and chin points and position the template on these two in order to locate the position of the angle and the condyle. This demonstrated that the opening movement is not hinge-like, but rather one which could occur only with a progressive change in position of the axis of rotation of the entire bone. The area of least movement is not at the condyle but in the mid-ramal region around the opening of the mandibular canal, the portal entry of the main blood and nerve supply of the bone. The figure also shows that the condyle has passed forward of the articular tubercle and entered the infratemporal fossa, a position in which at that time the jaw was generally considered to be dislocated.

Dissections led Chissin to announce that there were two heads to the external pterygoid muscle, superior and inferior. It had long been known that the muscle had attachment to the bone of the anterior surface of the neck of the condyle and to the capsular ligament above this at the level of the meniscus. He demonstrated that the two heads were separated by fascia. This has been verified by others, and the superior head has received the name of the "sphenomeniscus muscle." Later studies by others using methods that had meanwhile become available, such as cephalometric roentgenography, cineradiography, laminography, and electromyography, have substantiated the main conclusions of Chissin.

If the mandible opened like a simple hinge, one would expect an accompanying downward and backward rotation of the chin. This would be accompanied by similar movements of the hyoid bone, tongue, larynx, and pharynx, all of which are ultimately suspended from it in front. Such a movement would result in a shutting off of the airway. That they do not do so can be attributed to the marked adaptations that have occurred coincident to the attainment of vertical posture (Fig. 11d).

Reference has been made previously to certain skeletal changes that have accompanied the evolutionary change to an upright stance, such as the shortening of the muzzle and the outward flaring of the lower border of the mandible. Attention also has been called to the increase in mandibular height and to the balling up of the tongue. All of these have provided more room in back of the face and in the pharyngeal area, making it possible for muscles to assume the role played by gravity in horizontally oriented animals. The forward movement

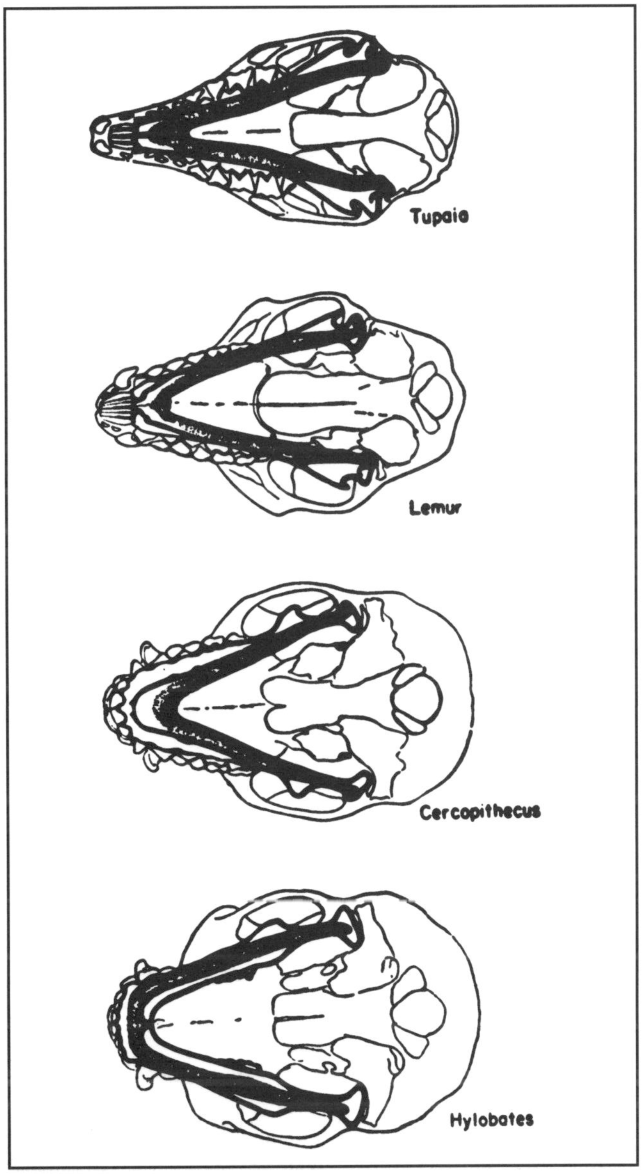

Fig. 11d. Change in position of foramen magnum with upright posture.

of the condyle by the external pterygoid reduces the impact of the backward swing of the mandible into the pharyngeal area during mouth opening, contributing greatly to the avoidance of respiratory embarrassment.

Maintenance of the Position of the Mandible

In the course of investigations on the normal and abnormal growth of the human head that have been carried on since 1932 in the Department of Orthodontics at the University of Illinois at Chicago College of Dentistry, there has been a constant recurrence of certain observations pertaining to the position of the mandible. These findings cause speculations as to the control of the position of this bone. Periodically the interest of the dental profession has been aroused to the point of controversy over such questions as the possibilities and limitations of full mouth reconstruction to raise the bite or otherwise alter mandibular position.

A review of the literature confirms the impression that there have been conflicting schools of thought in regard to the effect of the mandible concerning losses in vertical dimension through either attrition or extraction of teeth.

On the one hand, there were those who held to one or more of the following:

I. Such losses cause the mandible to assume a new relation to the maxilla. This new relation may be characterized by a protrusive drifting of the bone or a decrease in the vertical height of the face between nose and chin with the resulting falling in of the lips.

II. The loss of the "stopping" action of the teeth permits the masseter and internal pterygoid muscles to exert an unopposed pull on the angle of the mandible. This tension will presumably gradually flatten the angle and the neck of the condyles, causing a lengthening of the bone with consequent projection of the chin.

III. These changes of position in the condyle might and frequently do give rise to the so-called syndrome of Costen, the major symptoms of which are clicking noises, deafness, and joint pain of varying degrees.

On the other side of the question were opinions by men whose views were opposed to one or more of those points.

Heilman and Weinberger both expressed their disbelief that that mandibular angle flattened following the loss of teeth. Neiswonger and Gillis maintained that the rest position was a result of an equilibrium between the levator and depressor muscles running to the mandible and that in such a resting position the mandibular teeth were completely out of contact with the maxillary teeth. Tench and Mershon both pointed out that muscle tissue would probably limit the extent to which any bite could be raised.

It should be pointed out that most of the demonstrations purporting to show changes in the mandibular angle following loss of teeth had been made on series of dried skulls, in spite of the fact that any study of the human head quickly reveals such a great range of variability in each of its characteristics that such an approach to these questions is scientifically untenable. No series of skulls representing one age range can be compared to those representing a different age range to evaluate differences due to age or to changes in function. In a like manner, it is unsafe to rely solely on one's impressions when viewing living patients, regardless of how striking some apparent differences may seem. Nothing short of exact measurements will reveal what actually has taken place. Needless to say, it is even more unreliable to base conclusions on comparisons of the subjective reactions of one patient with those of another.

The studies of this problem, which will be described here, were conducted by means of roentgenographic cephalometry, which permits taking identical and accurate records of the same individual over long periods of time. The sample studied was a group of about 60 patients who reported to the prosthetic department of the dental school with various problems which called for artificial restorations. These included crown and bridge work as well as partial and full dentures.

Cephalometric roentgenograms were taken when the patient was first seen, and before any extractions were performed or impressions taken. In positioning the patients for those radiographs they were told to relax, and no reference was made to teeth. They were asked to swallow, and an x-ray exposure was then made about two seconds later. In cases requiring extraction, a second film was made just prior to the taking of the impression. All cases were radiographed once more immediately after dentures were inserted. These patients were called at quarterly and semiannual intervals thereafter for additional roentgenograms, both with the dentures in place and with the mouth empty.

Serial study of these cases soon made it apparent that the loss of teeth was not causing any change in the rest position of the mandible. However, wide differences were seen in the effect of extraction on different people. In some, the loss of teeth was followed by no great change; in others, the face from nose to chin seemed to collapse into the nutcracker pattern that has been held to present senility. When the reason for this difference was sought, it was found that those patients who seemed to be closing down were actually not holding the mandible in any different position, but instead they were showing the effects of more rapid alveolar resorption. Furthermore, such resorption affected not only the height of the process, but its thickness as well. The labial plate seemed to suffer equally with the crest, so that the lips were robbed not only of the support of the teeth but also that of the alveolar process. In several cases a loss of five millimeters (5 mm) in height and equal losses in thickness were demonstrated.

Facial change followed extraction of the incisors in one of these cases. The lips dropped inward because of loss of lingual support, and this made the chin appear to be more prominent. This type of facial change has frequently been ascribed to a decrease in the vertical dimension, yet in this case the tracing of the edentulous x-ray shows an actual increase in the vertical dimension. This was to be expected, since this patient had been instructed to close the teeth together during the original exposure, while the film taken after extraction was made with the mandible at physiologic rest. The rest position was confirmed in a radiograph made one month later.

In a number of the cases examined, the bite had been opened by dentures, so these reontgenograms with dentures in place revealed an increase in height over that which would have been indicated by the rest position. In all of these cases except one, the alveolar process underwent sufficient resorption to not only permit the mandible to return to its position of physiologic rest, but also to provide a freeway space as well. In one case, the opening of the bite had been successfully maintained for one year; a fact we can explain only on the basis of a high degree of accommodation or failure to detect closure beyond the rest position in the original radiograph.

Two typical cases in which the bite was opened by means of full dentures will be reported in detail. Neither had been subjected to recent extraction, so the preliminary resorption that follows extraction had already taken place. Case 30 was that of a woman age 52. The total face height with the mandible at rest was one hundred seven millimeters (107 mm). This rest position measurement was repeated twice, with subsequent readings of one hundred six point five millimeters (106.5 mm) and one hundred seven millimeters (107 mm). The total face height with the dentures in place and in occlusion, however, was one hundred eight point five millimeters (108.5 mm). Since a freeway space of two point five millimeters (2.5 mm) to three millimeters (3 mm) is considered to be the normal condition, we should add this to the one point five millimeters (1.5 mm) increase over rest position, for a total bite opening of four point five millimeters (4.5 mm). Change occurred in the facial height of this patient over a period of one year and four months. The dentures are in place, with the mandible in the physiologic rest position, and the chart indicates the total face height is now one hundred six point five millimeters (106.5 mm). Freeway space of two point five millimeters (2.5 mm) exists, so that with the denture in occlusion the face height is only one hundred four millimeters (104 mm).

Another case was that of a woman age 53. Physiologic rest position yielded a face height of one hundred eleven point five millimeters (111.5 mm), a reading that was confirmed by two other radiographs. The bite had been opened about six millimeters (6 mm). In the 13 months following denture placement a considerable amount of resorption of the underlying bone occurred. This permitted the bite to close until the mandible had regained its rest position and a freeway space of two millimeters (2 mm) had been established.

The partial denture cases were similarly illuminating. Here it was found that when the bite had been raised by such restorations, the mandible returned to its normal position even though this necessitated the depression of abutment teeth. Opportunity was not provided to examine a full-mouth reconstruction in which all of the teeth had been built up with crowns.

This investigation, plus those of normal, growing individuals seemed to support the following points:

I. The form and proportions of the human mandible are determined at a very early age, and once established, do not change.

II. The position of the mandible in relation to the rest of the face and head is an integral part of the pattern of the individual, and just as unchangeable as its form.

III. The presence or absence of teeth has little if any bearing on the form of the mandible, exclusive of the alveolar process.

IV. The presence or absence of teeth has little if any bearing on the rest position of the mandible, which is always such that the teeth are out of occlusion to a greater or lesser degree.

V. The rest position of the mandible is the result of a complex muscular coordination existing between the post-cervical muscles and those groups lying anteriorly which are concerned with the functions of mastication, respiration, deglutition, and speech. Acting as a unit they maintain the balanced posture of the head.

VI. The proportions of the face, so far as vertical height is concerned, are constant throughout life.

VII. The mean nasal height is forty three percent (43%) of total face height.

VIII. The Costen syndrome is not the result of a new position assumed by the mandible through loss of dental height, but rather is induced by over-closure of the mandible *in function*. It can be explained more logically on the basis of neuromuscular rather than mechanical functions.

IX. If the mandible is opened by artificial restorations to a position encroaching on the freeway space and physiologic rest position, it will return to its preordained position through an accommodation of the alveolar process by resorption or by depression of the abutment teeth.

Reading list:

Du Brul, E. Lloyd, and Sicher, Harry. *The Adaptive Chin.* Springfield, IL: Charles C. Thomas Publishers, 1954.

Steindler, Arthur. *Mechanics of normal and pathological locomotion in man*. Springfield, IL, and Baltimore, MD: Charles C. Thomas Publishers, 1935.

12.

Muscle Physiology of Head and Neck Region: Movement of Parts

Muscular Activity in Mouth Opening

One of the best examples of muscular coordination can be seen in mouth opening. Beginning with a resting position of the mandible, that is, with all of the muscles in a state of equilibrium, the external pterygoid begins to contract. This would, of course, result in a straight forward movement of the mandible were it not for the slope of the articular eminence which deflects the bone downward. Any downward movement would lead to increased tension in the remaining three muscles of the masticatory group, viz., masseter, internal pterygoid, and temporal, and as we have seen previously, such a tendency is offset by a reciprocal inhibition of those muscles.

But the downward movement of the mandible would also result in a dropping of the hyoid bone, together with those structures that are suspended from it (larynx, trachea, and pharynx). X-ray investigations have shown that such dropping does not occur, however, with the hyoid tending to remain at a constant level, although moving slightly backward. This means that tension is built up in the suprahyoid group in order to maintain the position of the hyoid. In accomplishing this, tension is naturally exerted on the anterior points of attachment of these muscles, all of which lie close to the symphysis of the mandible. Only in this manner, and to a certain degree, do the suprahyoid muscles contribute to mouth opening. The main source of power for this act is the external pterygoid.

Protrusive and Lateral Movements

Protrusive movements of the mandible are brought about almost exclusively by the external pterygoid and are always accompanied by a downward movement of the condyles on the eminentia articularis. This is a transitory type of movement which results in a disarticulating of the posterior teeth. What occurs at the front of the jaws depends on the state of contraction of the muscles of mastication. If these are inhibited, the mouth opens due to the downward and backward drag at the symphysis. If they are caused to contract slightly the incisor teeth are brought into contact, or the lowers may even pass in front of the uppers. This is the type of stroke employed in incising.

In lateral movements such as those employed in the mastication of food, the mandible operates in arcs in three planes of space. There is, of course, a certain amount of hinge action when the mouth opens, with the center of rotation located approximately in the middle of the condylar head. This represents movements in the sagittal plane. Movement in the horizontal plane is brought about by the unilateral contraction of the lateral pterygoid muscle, which pulls the head of the condyle on the *nonfunctioning* side forward while the opposite condyle remains in its fossa or may even move slightly backward. Movement in the frontal plane is unavoidable with any forward movement of the condyle because of the articular eminence. With unilateral forward movement the condyle on the nonfunctioning side is pulled to a lower level than that of the functioning side, so that the mandible is caused to rock in the frontal plane with the center of rotation in the head of the condyle of the functioning side.

Since the teeth are not habitually in contact when the individual is relaxed, it follows that they can have no influence on jaw movements until the mandible begins to travel from this resting position to occlusion. If, however, a tooth is in such a position that it does not permit smooth closing, the mandible usually will be deflected to a greater or lesser degree to avoid trauma on the offending tooth.

Deviation of the mandible from a straight path of either opening or closing also can be brought about by a number of joint conditions. A paralysis of the fifth nerve on one side will make it impossible for the external pterygoid muscle to advance the condyle on that side, and the mandible will deviate toward that side as the mouth is opened. A fracture of the neck of the condyle will operate in a similar manner, as will also partial ankylosis and extreme inflammatory reactions.

Movement in the frontal plane is unavoidable with forward movement of one condyle because of the articular eminence. With unilateral forward movement of the condyle on the nonfunctioning side, it is pulled to a lower level than that of the functioning side as it slides over the articular eminence so that the mandible is caused to rock in the frontal plane with the center of rotation in the head of the condyle of the opposite (functioning) side. This was demonstrated by Drake, who placed an orthodontic band on a lower incisor after soldering a vertical pin to its labial surface. Frontal cineradiograms were taken while the subject chewed gum. The film was enlarged by projection, and each frame was traced. Superposition of the tracing on points common to all of the extreme limits of movement yielded the findings.

There is at least one condition in which the mandibular midline does not coincide with that of the maxilla in both the rest and/or closed mouth position, but corrects itself as the mouth opens. This occurs with the development of a tumor in the glenoid fossa. As its mass increases, the tumor pushes the condyle out of the fossa and the midline of the mandible gradually is positioned further and further toward the opposite side. When the mouth opens in such a case, only the condyle on the normal side travels forward, tending to match the forward position of the opposite side and correct the midline.

The Effects of Muscle Tension on Fractured Bones

Bearing in mind that muscles are constantly under tension and that they will immediately shorten if given the opportunity, we can check the correctness of our ideas on muscle functions by observing the behavior of bone fragments following fracture. A moment's thought reveals that there are three areas of muscle attachment on the mandible and that the stresses operating on each are in different directions. Thus, at the condyle, there is a forward pull exerted by the external pterygoid; the rest of the ramus is under the influence of the masseter, temporal, and internal pterygoid, the mean pull of which is in an upward and forward direction; and the symphysis, where the suprahyoid muscles exert a downward and backward pull.

In a unilateral fracture of the condyle neck the condyle is rotated forward and upward by the pull of the external pterygoid, and the ramus moves slightly backward because of the unopposed pull of the temporalis. Aside from this latter change no other alteration is apparent in the position of the mandible until the mouth is opened. Now the external pterygoid on the uninjured side brings the condyle forward without a similar movement taking place on the injured side, and the jaw is seen to swing toward the side of the fracture.

Fractures at the junction of the body and ramus witness an upward and forward rotation of the ramus, induced by the pull of the masticatory group, while the body tends to drop because of the tensions from the suprahyoid group.

Bilateral fractures which leave the anterior part of the body free are characterized by a downward and backward displacement of that part. Such fractures can be highly dangerous because this area also supplies attachment for those muscles which hold the tongue forward, and without such anchorage the tongue is apt to choke the patient.

Muscle Function in Facial Fractures

Fractures of the coronoid process are rare. They would be expected to retract the process alone, upward and backward into the temporal fossa. Fractures at the junction of the body and ramus result in an upward and forward rotation of the ramus induced by the pull of the masseter and internal pterygoid, while the body tends to be drawn down by the tensions from the suprahyoid group, especially the mylohyoid.

The degree of displacement of the fragments in bilateral fractures of the body of the mandible depends on the force and direction of the original blow as well as on the muscle tensions operating afterward, and both may be modified by impaction at the sites of the fractues. If the fragments do not impact and the fractures are toward the front of the mandible (lateral-canine areas), there is danger of choking. The hyoid bone, which is the foundation for the tongue, as well as the tongue itself, both are suspended in front from the genial tubercles on the internal surface of the symphysis. With the release of their tension, the entire tongue is drawn downward and backward against the airway.

13. Muscle Physiology of Head and Neck Region: Internal

Internal Musculature

In a previous chapter, attention was drawn to the fact that the head was positioned on a flexible column by the balanced tensions of groups of muscles together with gravity and, further, that certain of the areas of attachment of these muscles were movable. These parts (cranium, mandible, hyoid, and shoulder girdle) must, in addition, act as the bases of action for other muscle groups having quite different and highly specialized functions. These groups might be thought of as lying internally to those which control the relationships of the skeletal parts. They are:

The Tongue

The tongue can be thought of as a muscular mass which almost completely fills the oral cavity from birth onward. Its intrinsic musculature, which has no bony attachment, can alter its form since it is disposed in the three planes of space. Contraction of the transversalis narrows and elongates it while the verticalis flattens, broadens, and lengthens it. The superior longitudinalis curls the tip upward, the inferior longitudinalis curls the tip downward, while the combined action of the two tends to shorten the organ and make it thicken. None of its intrinsic muscles can affect its position.

This muscle mass is suspended in a manner not unlike that of the mandible and hyoid bones, but now those suspended parts must be considered as fixed points of anchorage. The genohyoglossus is a fan-shaped muscle arising from the superior genial tubercle on the inner surface of the symphysis of the mandible, its lower fibers running straight downward and backward to the hyoid bone and its other fibers being disposed fan-like from the hyoid bone to the tip of the tongue. This is the muscle that holds the tongue forward. The styloglossus arises, as its name implies, from the styloid process of the temporal bone and runs downward, forward, and medialward to insert into the sides and dorsum of the tongue. It suspends the tongue from above and in back. The palatoglossus or anterior pillar of the fauces is in a position to aid in tongue suspension, but its major function is probably that of sealing the mouth as a sphincter to prevent the return of food to that cavity from the pharynx. Completing the extrinsic group is the hyoglossus, which runs upward and forward to the side of the tongue from the superior surface of the greater cornu of the hyoid bone. This muscle, although undoubtedly modifying the tongue's position by transmitting part of the weight of the larynx to that organ, is of greater significance as a contributor to deglutition, as we shall see later.

Thus we realize that the tongue is completely controlled by muscles which run to it from outside points, one at the midline of the mandible and two from widely separate cranial points. This is a three-point suspension and the disposition of the three points, plus the tonus of the suspensory muscles, determine the resting position of the tongue.

The Soft Palate

The basic framework of the soft palate is an aponeurosis or connective tissue sheet which is attached along the full extent of the posterior edge of the hard palate. Its position, or level, at any instant is dependent on its functioning at the time. Thus, in normal quiet respiration, it hangs down in contact with the dorsum of the tongue, leaving the air passage behind it open. In this position its controlling musculature is in equilibrium. Its muscles are four in number, viz., levator veli palatini, tensor veli palatini, palatoglossus, and palatopharyngeus. The first two run to it from above, the latter two from below.

The tensor veli palatini is a triangularly-shaped sheet of muscle, the base of the triangle being its attachment which extends from the spina angularis of the sphenoid along the cartilaginous external auditory tube, forward and medially to the wall of the pharynx. Here its margin follows the wall of that organ until it reaches the level of the hamulus of the medial pterygoid plate, where it becomes tendinous and enters the pharynx to spread out and mingle its fibers with those of the aponeurosis of the soft palate. Its vertical contraction is transformed into a straight lateral pull by its pulley-like change of direction at the hamulus and it pulls the soft palate tense, thus effecting a prolongation of the palate to the postpharyngeal wall and a closing-off of the nasopharynx.

The levator veli palatini arises from the tip of the petrous element of the temporal bone and is thus closer to the midline than is the tensor. It runs over the superior border of the superior constrictor pharyngeus, downward and somewhat forward, to spread out in the soft palate. By its upward and backward pull it assists the tensor to raise the palate, but in addition it also domes that structure so that it conforms to the form of the hard palate.

The glossopharyngeus muscle runs a curved course from the under surface of the palatal musculature to the side and dorsum of the tongue. With the uvula, these paired muscles hug the tongue back against themselves to prevent the return of food into the mouth once it has passed the anterior pillar.

The pharyngopalatinus is usually described as running from the musculature of the underside of the soft palate, down the side of the pharynx to spread out in its lateral wall. However, there is another school of thought that holds that this muscle is a very old sphincter which is present in birds and many lower animals in which the airway and upper gut are disposed in a horizontal manner. In these there is a definite sphincter running from the posterior end of the hard palate, around an opening, to become continuous with the dorsal side of the gut. This opening receives the upper end of the airway, an extended epiglottis, which is grasped by the sphincter and held within the nose except when the animal is eating. During this act the windpipe is withdrawn and the sphincter closes the opening into the nose. According to this school, the palatopharyngeus muscle in humans performs a somewhat similar function. Arching backward and downward from close to the midline of the soft palate it follows the upper margin of the superior constrictor and acts as a sphincter of the upper end of the pharynx, throwing its margin into a prominent ridge which is called Passavant's bar.

The Pharynx

The pharynx is the upper, dilated part of the gut and lies just back and below the mouth cavity. Its intrinsic musculature consists of its three constrictors which extend from under the cranium to the esophagus, the superior extending down inside the middle constrictor which in turn extends downward inside the inferior, which in turn becomes continuous with the esophagus. Throughout the entire course of these three pairs of muscles they are attached at the midline above, to the pharyngeal tubercle of the basi-occipital and in back to the precervical fascia. They are hence largely fixed. That is not the case for the anterior attachments. The anterior margins of the superior constrictors take attachment from the lower one-half of the medial pterygoid plate and from the pterygomandibular raph, which runs from its hamulus to the posterior end of the mylohyoid line on the internal surface of the mandible opposite the last molar tooth.

Note: Since the buccinator muscle takes its posterior attachment from that same raph, there is a continuous muscle sheet running from the base of the cranium and the vertebral column, forward and around the dental arches.

The middle constrictors have their anterior attachments on the stylohyoid ligament, the lesser cornu and superior surface of the greater cornu, of the hyoid bone. From here their fibers run both upward and downward as they proceed posteriorly to their precervical attachment at the midline. This is a diamond-shaped muscle when viewed from the back.

The inferior constrictors take their anterior attachment from the posterolateral margins of the thyroid and cricoid cartilages of the larynx, the superior fibers coursing upward around the inferior borders of the middle constrictors, and the inferior fibers running horizontally, hence parallel, to those of the esophagus. Thus it can be seen that the tongue, epiglottis, and larynx form the anterior wall of the pharynx.

This muscular tube is suspended on the sides by three muscles: the palatopharyngeus, already described; the stylopharyngeus, from the styloid process of the temporal bone; and the salpingopharyngeus from the torus at the inner end of the Eustachean tube. However, the pharynx derives most of its support from the hyoid bone and from its fascial attachment to the cervical vertebrae. Except during the taking of food the pharynx is almost collapsed anteroposteriorly at its lower end, and even at the upper laryngeal level it is not fully distended.

The Larynx

The laryngopharyngeal mechanism must be viewed as a valve that became necessary when the air intake was switched from the gills, which were ventral to the gut, to the nose, which is dorsal. This brought about a crossing of the food and air channels. Our interest in the larynx lies in our need to understand the functions of deglutition and speech, but principally the former.

The framework of the larynx consists of two major cartilages, the thyroid and cricoid, which constitute most of its bulk and contain within their boundaries the other cartilages, viz., the epiglottis, the two arytenoids, two corniculate, and two cuneiform. It is these smaller cartilages that play the major role in the valve action, however.

The thyroid cartilage, largest of the laryngeal cartilages, consists of two large laminae, joined at the midline anteriorly, with their posterior margins extending superiorly and inferiorly in cornua. The entire superior margin of the cartilage gives origin to a sheet of dense fibrous connective tissue which runs upward *inside* the hyoid bone and takes attachment to the entire superior margin of that bone. This connective tissue sheet is strengthened at the midline and at the posterior limits, between the end of the greater cornu of the hyoid and the tip of the superior cornu of the thyroid, by additional fibers; this makes them ligaments. This arrangement makes a virtual unit of the hyoid bone and the upper end of the larynx, so that the latter must share in the movements of the former.

The cricoid cartilage lies just below and partly within the lower margin of the thyroid. Shaped like a signet ring, the body articulates on its sides with the medial surface of the inferior cornua beneath the lower margin of the thyroid laminae. This type of articulation between the two cartilages makes possible a slight rocking motion of the cricoid.

The arytenoid cartilages, two in number, sit on the upper margin of the cricoid cartilage and are held in this position by articular capsules which enclose facets on the two approximating surfaces. These cartilages are pyramidal in shape, but their four surfaces are not equal. Their bases, which face the cricoid, are slightly concave, as are also their posterior surfaces. Their approximating surfaces are almost parallel throughout their extent although also slightly concave. The fourth surface faces anteriorly, laterally, and upward, is slightly convex, and presents a faint ridge running in a curved direction from the apex downward and forward to the midline termination. Like any pyramid, each of the arytenoids has three base angles. That at the posterior medial junction is regular but the other two, i.e., the posterior lateral and anteromedial, are accentuated with processes which have to do with function. The posterolateral is called "the muscular process" and gives attachment to the posterior and lateral cricoarytenoid muscles. The anteromedial is called "the vocal process" and gives attachment to both the vocal ligament and ventricular fold. It is sufficient for our interests to state that the posterior and lateral cricoarytenoid muscles, running to the same processes on the arytenoid cartilages from directions at right angles to each other, cause rotations of the arytenoid on the body of the cricoid. The rotation of the posterior muscle carries the two vocal processes apart and thus opens the glottis, while the lateral pair rotates them toward each other, closing the glottis.

Our major interest in the larynx lies in its function of closing the airway against the ingress of food during the act of deglutition. This is largely the role of the internal cartilages, viz., the arytenoids, the cuneiforms, the corniculates, and the epiglottis.

Surmounting the apex of the arytenoid cartilages which have already been described are two small cartilaginous nodules, the corniculate and cuneiform cartilages. The epiglottis is a leaf-like cartilage which extends well above the hyoid bone and lies against the base of the tongue to which it is loosely attached by a midline and two lateral connective tissue and membrane folds. Its lower end is attached to the internal surface of the thyroid cartilage, at the midline and about half way between upper and lower borders, by an elastic ligament. Somewhat above this attachment the posterior aspect of the epiglottis presents a marked midline swelling the tubercle.

Controlling all of these cartilages is a muscle, the arytenoepiglottic, which acts as a sphincter. This muscle arises laterally on the base of the arytenoid cartilage, and runs upward and medialward to pass around the apex of the opposite arytenoid. The corniculate and cuneiform cartilages lie within the fold of tissue which encloses the muscle after it has passed the apex of the arytenoid. Continuing in an upward but now forward direction, the arytenoepiglottic fold passes along the side of the epiglottis just below the level of the tubercle and takes attachment to the *anterior* surface of that cartilage.

If the location of this fold of tissue, together with its associated muscle, has been visualized, it is not difficult to understand its action. Its course around the apex of the arytenoid would tip that cartilage medially and forward, as well as tend to approximate the two paired cartilages which lie within its folds. Its attachment to the epiglottis would pull the lower part, or tubercle, backward and downward into contact with the previously mentioned pairs. In this movement the upper part of the epiglottis cannot share because of its attachment to the tongue. Thus, if there were no movement of the tongue or hyoid bone together with the larynx, which is suspended from the latter, food would pass from the dorsum of the tongue backward and downward over the posterior surface of the epiglottis and in turn over the corniculate and cuneiform cartilages and posterior surfaces of the arytenoids. Actually, however, because of extensive movement of the tongue and hyoid bone, such contact with food does not take place except in the case of the epiglottis. The rest of the larynx is pulled well forward and upward by the geniohyoid muscles, and the tongue rolls back. Such forward movement of the larynx opens the pharynx because of the attachment of the constrictors to the laryngeal cartilages and hyoid bone, and thus the sphincter muscle with its enclosed nodules of cartilage comes to lie in a vertical plane so that food could only enter it if there is a sudden inspiration of air.

From all that has been said about the muscles of the head and neck, it can be seen that the apparent stability of the various parts is a result solely of the interplay of muscular forces. Actually, the relation of the head to the vertebral column (itself a highly unstable structure) is a precarious teetering of a globe-like structure on a pole. Dorsally, a continuous group of muscles runs from base of cranium to shoulder girdle and vertebral column, and one side balances the other. Ventrally, the same connection between cranium and base of anchorage is broken into three sets of independent muscles which, in addition to controlling the posture of the head, must each perform its own distinctive function as well as enable the other groups to perform theirs by the stabilization of parts.

The Musculature of the Hyoid Bone

Suspended entirely by muscles which run to it from many directions, the hyoid bone, like a man in a parachute, is positioned at rest by an equilibrium of their tensions. In function it acts to coordinate the activities of those two most vital systems, the respiratory and the digestive. To serve its dual roles it must alternate between intense states of activity and firm stability. In addition, it must adjust instantly to the changes of all influences that might impinge on it. As has been pointed out, gravity is one of those influences, particularly in humans.

Longitudinal studies on large numbers of individuals have shown that the hyoid bone remains at a level which varies between the lower third of the third and the upper third of the fourth cervical vertebra; it is stable within the individual. As the vertebrae grow in height, the hyoid bone descends vertically with them and the muscles running to it from in back (stylohyoid, posterior digastric) lengthen proportionately, maintaining its stability.

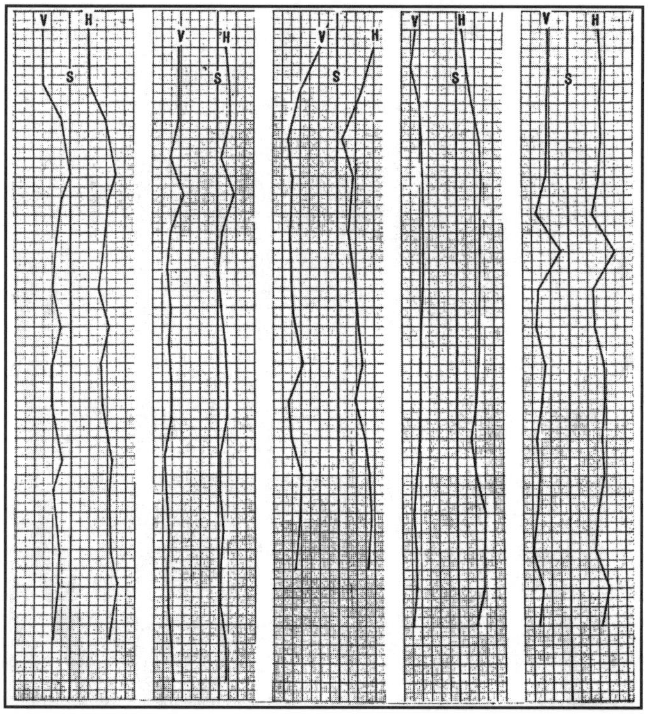

Fig. 13a. Diagrams of five cases studied showing synchronous movement of hyoid in cervical flexion when reference points are brought to the same horizontal level.

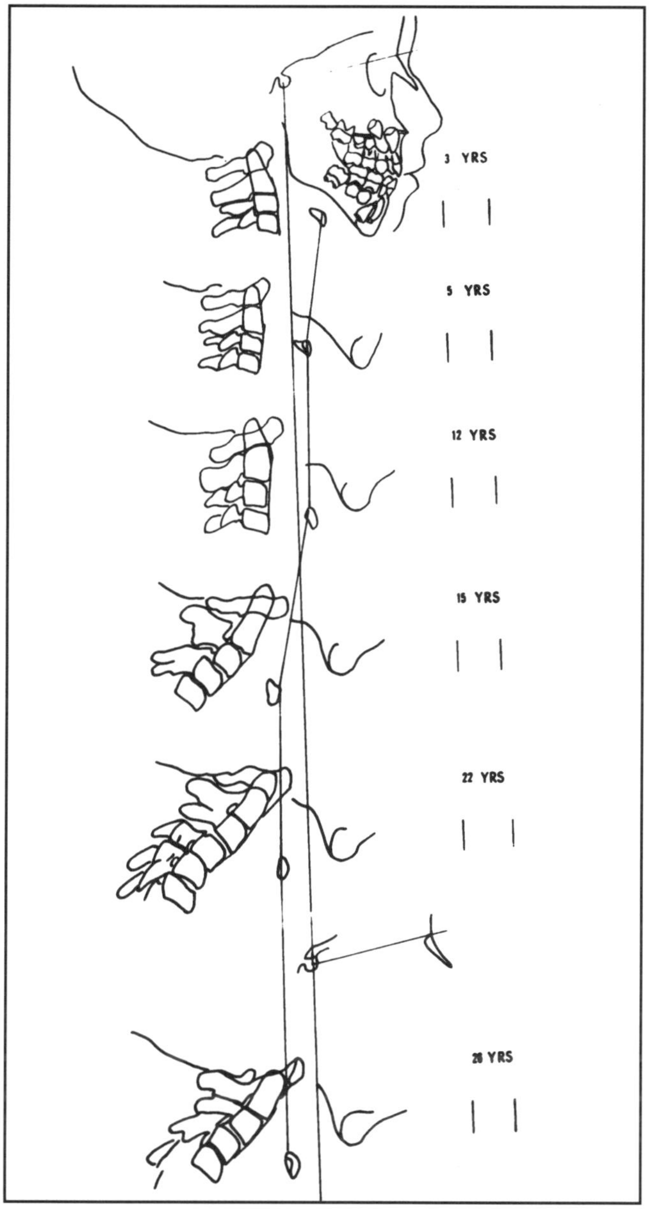

Fig. 13b. Tracings of serial cephalometric roentgenograms of a patient who suffered from rheumatoid arthritis beginning in childhood and experienced progressive backward movement of the chin and hyoid bone. The vertical parallel lines on the right represent the shortest distance between cervical vertebrae and hyoid bone assuring airway maintenance.

Growth Behavior of the Hyoid Bone*

King studied the growth of the pharynx in relation to certain cranial, facial, and vertebral bony points. Durzo, using similar methods, sought to determine if there were any changes in the position of the hyoid bone coincident with the vocal changes in males at adolescence. On an all-male

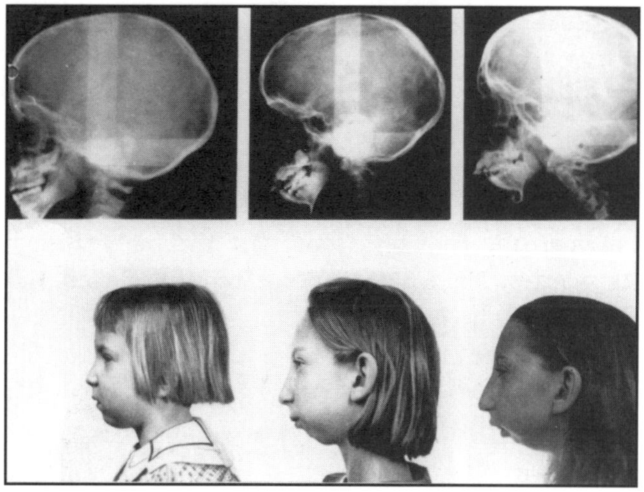

Fig. 13c.

sample of serial cephalometric roentgenograms he traced the details shown in Fig. 13a. He constructed the Frankfurt horizontal and a vertical plane through S for references. Additional lines were drawn to RHS, the highest point on the silhouette of the symphysis of the mandible. This last point represented the genial tubercles. The two resulting lines represented the posterior and anterior suprahyoid muscles respectively. RAS represents the most anterior part on the axis.

Because flexions of the cervical vertebrae had occurred during exposure of some of the cephalograms, points RVS and RHS did not follow a straight downward course parallel with RSS, but, significantly, remained parallel to each other. The anteroposterior dimension of the airway remained unchanged from the 3rd to the 17th year, as determined by measurements made at the shortest distance between the hyoid bone and the vertebrae. Failure of the mandible to move downward and forward with growth in a subject suffering an arrest of condylar development was shown to maintain her original airway dimension by a gradual increase of the tension in the anterior hyoid muscles (Fig. 13b and c).

*See Appendix II: Endnotes.

Reading list:

Durzo, Carmine. *Growth behavior of the Hyoid bone: a serial x-ray study.* Thesis (MS in orthodontia), University of Illinois, 1961.

14.
The Periodontal Ligament

The periodontal ligament is made up principally of the connective tissue which occupies the space between the root of a tooth and the bony wall of its socket. Transplantation of tooth germs has shown that it results from the orientation of elements of the mesenchyme of the dental sac. The mesenchyme surrounds the germ prior to the appearance of Hertwig's epithelial sheath and the beginning of root formation.

Root formation is accompanied by the start of eruption. A marked change occurs in the arrangement of the cellular elements of the undifferentiated mesenchyme. They become oriented to run from root to bone. There is a coarse layer adjacent to the bone and an inner, more loosely arranged zone next to the root. As bone and cementum begin to form at the respective ends of the fibers, a third layer of fibers appears between them. This has been given the name of Plexus Intermedius (Sicher), and is thought to be characteristic of rapid eruption. It is seen normally in the continuously growing incisors of rodents. In humans it becomes indistinguishable after occlusion has been attained. The nature of its functional activity is not known, however. It has been suggested that it is a zone of replacement of fibers, new fibers being formed and attached to those anchored to bone and to cementum as older intermediate fibers are eliminated. That some such activity must take place continually and not only during periods of rapid eruption is suggested by the observation that the fibers do not run directly from tooth to bone but in wavy courses that result in their intertwining.

The principle fibers of the periodontal ligament have been classified (Black, 1887) according to their apparent roles as resistors to the functional forces operating on the teeth. They are understood best if one considers them as suspensory devices counteracting functional forces by increases of tension. Viewed in this manner, it is apparent that pressure forces, such as those of mastication operating on teeth, are transmitted as tensions to the bone to which they are attached. However, there are fibers that act otherwise.

Beginning at the crest of the alveolus, the first is the free gingival group, the fibers of which pass occlusally from the cementum to the gingiva and support it. The transeptal fibers pass from their attachment in the cementum of one tooth to that of the next, and the alveolar crest fibers pass downward to the crest of the surrounding alveolar bone. These three groups, together with the fibers which encircle the crown and those of the fibrous mat which underlies the mucosa, keep the gingiva close to the tooth surface.

They are inextricably interwoven so as to prevent accurate separation into groups. Nevertheless, the functions they serve have long been recognized by the clinician as well as the microscopist. This complex has been known as the ligamentum circulare, or dental ligament, and its most conspicuous function is to keep the teeth together in their arches. However, the free gingival and alveolar crest elements serve important roles in the protection and support of the interproximal tissues. The alveolar crest group is the only one whose direction and course might suggest an eruption-restraining tension, but even this could be interpreted as a growth-stimulating tension on the crest, which seems more likely.

The fibers below the level of the crest are at first mainly horizontal in direction, but become increasingly oblique as they pass downward from the alveolar wall to the root. These are the main stress bearers of the forces of mastication. As pointed out in the lesson on root form, the effective resistance of any tooth to force put upon it is determined by the area of root surface available for the attachment of periodontal fibers. Since all functional forces operating on the teeth move in arcs, not in straight lines, it is self-evident that the direction of stress does not remain constant after the instant of impact; it changes continuously with the progress of the stroke. The multidirectional arrangement of the fibers, as shown in a horizontal microscopic section at the level of the crest of the alveolar border, as well as the wavy, curved course of the fibers themselves, convey an impression of limitless adaptability to withstand forces from all directions in that plane.

There has long been controversy over the manner in which a tooth moves when force is exerted upon it. Some maintain that it acts like a post in the ground, i.e., the ends move reciprocally in opposite directions, although not necessarily by the same amount. Others hold that the root end is the center of rotation, which reduces all tooth movements to tipping. Strangely enough, there is evidence enough to support both views. All orthodontists know how simple it is to tip a displaced tooth into position if there is no occlusal interference to such movement, and if the root end is approximately in its normal position.

Oppenheim's studies on apes (1910) revealed that the reaction to a periodically renewed force exerted by ligature traction occured first at the rim of the alveolus. In addition to this, he made the following observations: the periodontal ligament was compressed to 1/3 of its normal thickness almost the entire length of the root, but there was no thrombosis anywhere as claimed by Sandsted. There were small hemorrhages and some diapedesis of blood corpuscles through the vessel walls. Cell numbers were remarkably increased and staining reactions were normal. The characteristic directions of the fibers of the periodontal ligament were preserved unchanged and the fibers of the ligamentum circulare had suffered no disturbance.

There was fragmentation of the compact bone of the labial wall of the alveolus and its replacement by spicules of spongy bone, which sprang from the labial surfaces of the resorbing spicules and were oriented at right angles to the long axis of the tooth. All of the reactions diminished to a point 2/3 down the root below which the tissues appeared normal. This experiment was of 40-day duration, and Oppenheim assumed from it that if it had been continued for a longer period the changes would have extended to the apex. He expressed his convictions as follows: "The standpoint is not correct as held by many authors that the tooth represents a two-armed lever with its fulcrum at the alveolar border or at the middle of the root and that on labial movement of a tooth, for instance, there must be bone absorption at the labial alveolar border and also on the lingual side of the root end. The tooth represents a one-armed lever and the apex of the root serves as the pivot point or center of rotation. In the bone of immediate proximity to the root apex there were no changes observable."

In contrast to the findings resulting from the application of light "physiological" forces were those following the use of heavy forces. The labial compact bone was entirely unaltered, except that it was somewhat attenuated throughout. Osteoclasts on the side of pressure appeared only sporadically, and there was complete absence of signs of bone formation on the surface away from the tooth, with osteoblasts occurring only in scattered layers. No budding was visible on any bone surface. The periodontal ligament was 1/3 of its normal width, fibrous in appearance and markedly deficient in cells. The blood vessels appeared engorged or thrombosed. All of these signs bespeak a strangulation of blood supply.

The microscopic changes that might take place around the root of a tooth were of scant interest to the practicing orthodontist; his concern lay with the position of the crown. Tipping of teeth into position, which seemed to be indicated by Oppenheim's study, sometimes resulted in undue prominence of the incisors and Case, in 1895, sought to prevent this by employing separate arches at two levels of the tooth crown in order to employ double leverages. Similar unpleasant protrusions troubled Angle, and both men were controlling such protrusions by the extraction of premolars.

At the time the x-ray, or "skiagraph" as it was called, was rarely used in orthodontia and its use in routine record-taking was a decade in the future. It is not surprising therefore that the orthodontist had given little thought to the possibility that his procedures might have deleterious effects. Thus he was rudely shaken by a paper titled "A Preliminary Report of an Investigation of Apical Root Resorption of Permanent Teeth" by A.H. Ketcham in 1927. Ketcham had been one of Angle's followers who had adopted the ribbon arch and had surveyed a sample of his treated cases.

Ketcham's report completely diverted the attention of the investigators from tooth movement per se to root resorption, and the two came to be viewed as cause and effect. As might be expected, the ribbon arch came under heavy attack. Its strength and rigidity were held to exert "unphysiological forces," and these became the culprits in root resorption by consensus. They could not be exerted by such appliances as the lingual arch, whose forces acted through light springs gently pressing against the crowns of the tooth. Such appliances were held by their users to be physiologic in their action.

Bibliography covering these matters is too extensive for adequate treatment here, but the conglomeration of ideas, experimental materials and methods, conclusions, theories, and concepts requires that they be put in better perspective than is afforded by chronology alone. Principally, it is essential to recognize that many problems are presented, each of which may call for different attacks in order to reach narrower and, hopefully, sounder conclusions. The case in point is the lumping together of the studies of tooth movement and root resorption. What we think we know about each must first be noted before any attempt is made to consider them together.

Earlier, a cursory review was made of the structures of the periodontal ligament as it appears in texts of dental histology (Noyes, Schour, Sicher, Orban, Kronfeld). There is general agreement that it is in the nature of a suspensory network of bundles of collagen fibers running between the cementum of the tooth root and the alveolar bone, both of which it forms as the root grows. Forces operating on the crown are resisted by tensing of the fibers on the side receiving the force. The force is not exerted against taut fibers, but against fibers which run in curved courses and which are interwoven with others from which they are separated by blood and lymph vessels. These provisions allow for the small movements of individual teeth against their neighbors that results in interproximal wear, shown so strikingly in the heavy functioning teeth of aborigines. Such movements apparently cause no reaction in the bone, and the previous condition of the ligament is immediately restored when force is removed.

Most histologic studies of orthodontically induced tooth movement have been interpreted from the standpoint of the reactions of the alveolar bone around the tooth. Although these have yielded much valuable information, one can easily realize that the tooth movements can only be mediated through the periodontal ligament. It would be the first link in the chain of reaction. What occurs in it?

As has been noted elsewhere, those fiber-bundles that have been attached to the root of the tooth by cementoblasts are not the same fibers that are attached to alveolar bone by osteoblasts, i.e., neither set is continuous. Sicher (1923) introduced the term "plexus intermedius" to denote a zone between them where the free ends of both groups meet. Here they are thought to lie side by side in their ground substance bound by mucopolysaccarides (Furstman and Bernick, 1972, Fig. 14a). Steady tension on them of only short duration (less than two hours) results in a slackening of the chemical bonds between them and a spacing and sliding of the fibers.

How recovery takes place from such tension is not known, whether by reversal of the bonding process or by the elaboration of new fibers. That the latter unquestionably accompanies recovery was shown by Macapanpan (1954), who demonstrated a sharp increase of mitoses among the fibroblasts on the tension side of teeth of experimental rats.

The orthodontist can take advantage of the initial response noted above under certain circumstances. One of these is the crossbite in which a single tooth deflects the mandible into an abnormal anteroposterior or mediolateral occlusion. It is found most frequently in the incisor region where an upper central may close deeply behind the lower teeth. Handing the patient a mirror, he is asked to see how far in back of his upper front teeth he can close his lowers without assistance. If he demonstrated the ability to attain an edge-to-edge relation or one near it, the tooth can probably be tipped across the bite in a matter of minutes in the chair while prying labially on the tooth with a wooden tongue blade resting against the lower incisors. This procedure represents the application of one of the oldest mechanical principles used in orthodontia: the inclined plane. Highly effective, it is non-harmful because it is governed by the pain threshold of the patient. It is, however, quite limited in the extent and scope of its effectiveness.

Having passed beyond the stage of limited response and assuming the continuation of the operating force, it becomes necessary to examine the next link in the chain. This is the bone of the alveolus, from which the tooth is suspended by the fibers. It is at this level that the responses of bone become evident, and these have received the most attention by investigators. They are in general agreement that the very lightest force will elicit a response in living bone by the appearance of osteoblasts on the side of tension and osteoclasts on the opposite side. This poses a question of whether there is a state of tension in the periodontal ligament at all times, and if this tension is essential to maintain the bone. A force which would increase tension on one side would lead to a decrease of tension on the opposite side. Is it such a *release of tension* that initiates resorption, or is it pressure, as has always been claimed?

To attempt to answer this question, a band was formed on a lower central incisor of a well-developed male adult, whose lower incisors were spaced. Mesial and distal spurs were run from the band to just make contact with, but not to exert pressure against, the two adjacent teeth. The object was to note the behavior of the tooth when its independent resistance was shared with other teeth. Upon removal of the band after one week, the tooth was demonstrably less firm than its neighbors, although it attained its former stability in 24 hours.

Does this imply that a degree of tension is required to maintain "tone" in the fibers, as is the case in muscle?

Oppenheim's earliest study, and many of those that have followed, have revealed hyaline degeneration accompanying the narrowing of the periodontal ligament on the side of pressure, that is, opposite the side of tension. This is thought to be the result of reduced cellular activity due to diminished blood supply. Osteoclasts appear attacking the bone where the force is sufficiently attenuated to elicit their response.

The answer seems clear that the slightest forces that can be applied will induce the fastest responses in the tissues. The orthodontist tends to apply force according to the adage, "If a little is good, a whole lot must be better." This defeats his purpose, for while he may ultimately gain the movement he desires, he does so at the expense of the time it has taken to rebuild the areas of undermining resorption which heavy force has created.

It would seem from this that the orthodontist must begin to think of the tooth-jaw relation as something other than a post in a hole. Rather than thinking exclusively in terms of pressures, major attention should be directed toward tensions which are the main resisters of force: the fibers of the periodontal membrane. Only against a force operating in a straight gingival direction could it be conceivably possible to tense all the fibers of the ligament simultaneously. From any other direction, the force would give rise to resisting tensions at a point of resistance, viz., the fulcrum, but since functional forces such as those of mastication change continually during the stroke, so must the point of resistance continually change. All animal tissues are adapted to such "work and rest" cycles, and it is only when the cycle is disturbed that changes can be noted in them. It is this that makes the orthodontic movement of teeth possible.

Orthodontic movement is accomplished most simply by bringing to bear pressure or tension forces upon a tooth at a single point. This results in tipping of the tooth, as shown by Oppenheim. The earliest response takes place at the top of the alveolus on the tension side where spicules are built in line with the force. They are of osteoid tissue heavily beset with osteoblasts.

The process progresses apically as tension acts at lower and lower levels. On the side away from the tension, the wall of the alveolus facing the root is attacked by osteoclasts which undermine and fragment, while the surfaces of the alveolus away from the root present buds of osteoid tissue on which osteoblasts will deposit new bone.

It must be realized that the number of variables involved in the matter of tooth movement, not to mention the gradations within each, makes any dogmatic statement regarding it impossible. One can accept as a fact only that a tooth will move under the influence of a force brought to bear upon it. But beyond that, any statement regarding such matters as the precise site of initial response, location and nature of resistance, and optimal type and application of stimulation, i.e., steady or intermittent, must remain dependent upon the background, experience, and judgment of the operator.

Reading list:

Macapanpan, Luz Celis. *Early tissue changes flowing tooth movement in rats.* Thesis (MS in orthodontia), University of Illinois, 1952.

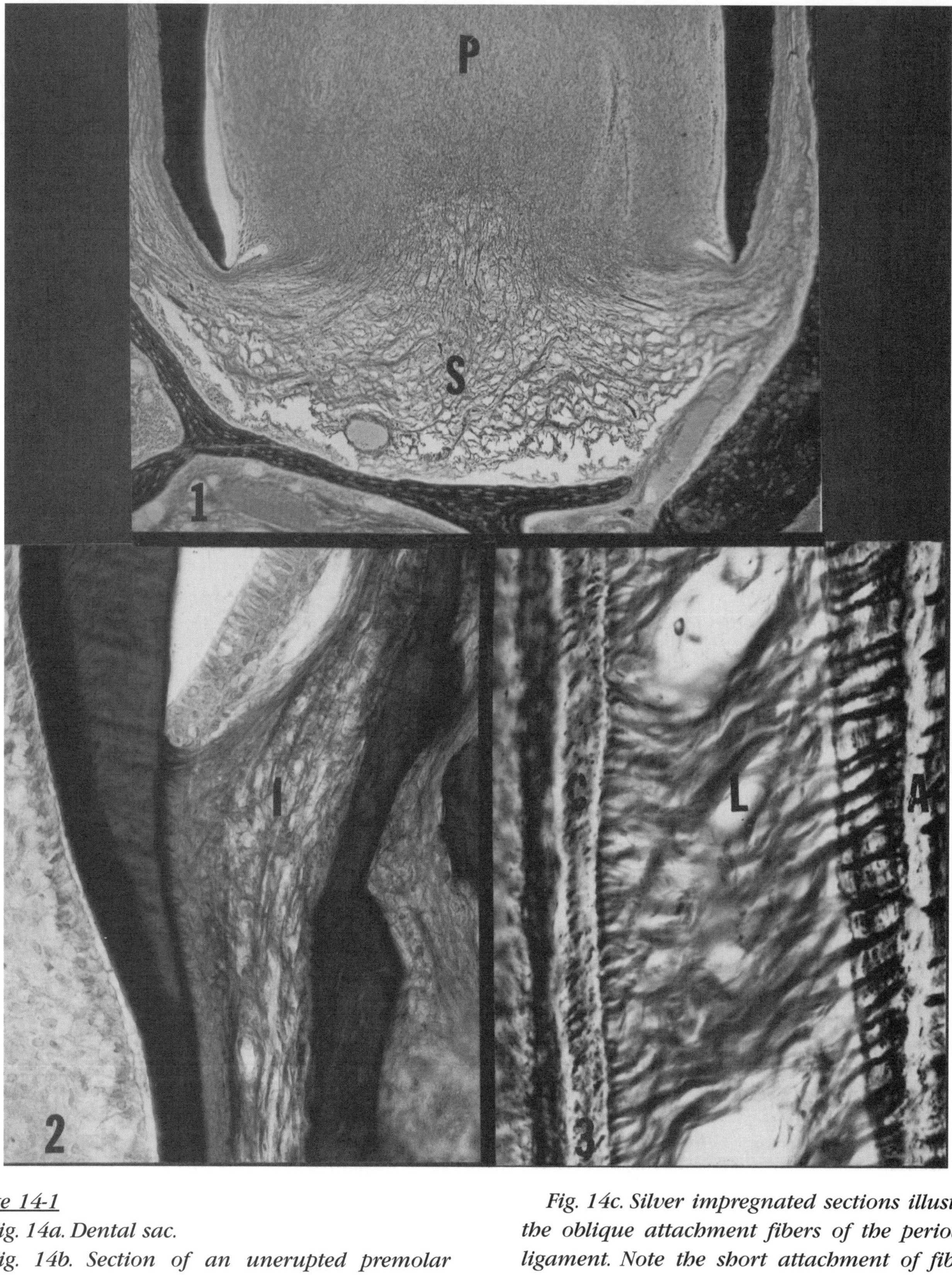

Plate 14-1

Fig. 14a. Dental sac.

Fig. 14b. Section of an unerupted premolar tooth illustrating the plexus intermedius. Note the short cemental and osseous fibers emerging from bone and cementum. The plexus intermedius consists of loose disorganized fibers.

Fig. 14c. Silver impregnated sections illustrating the oblique attachment fibers of the periodontal ligament. Note the short attachment of fibers at the cementum and the long Sharpey's fibers in the alveolar bone.

P-Pulp S-Dental Sac

1-Plexus Intermedius L-Periodontal Ligament

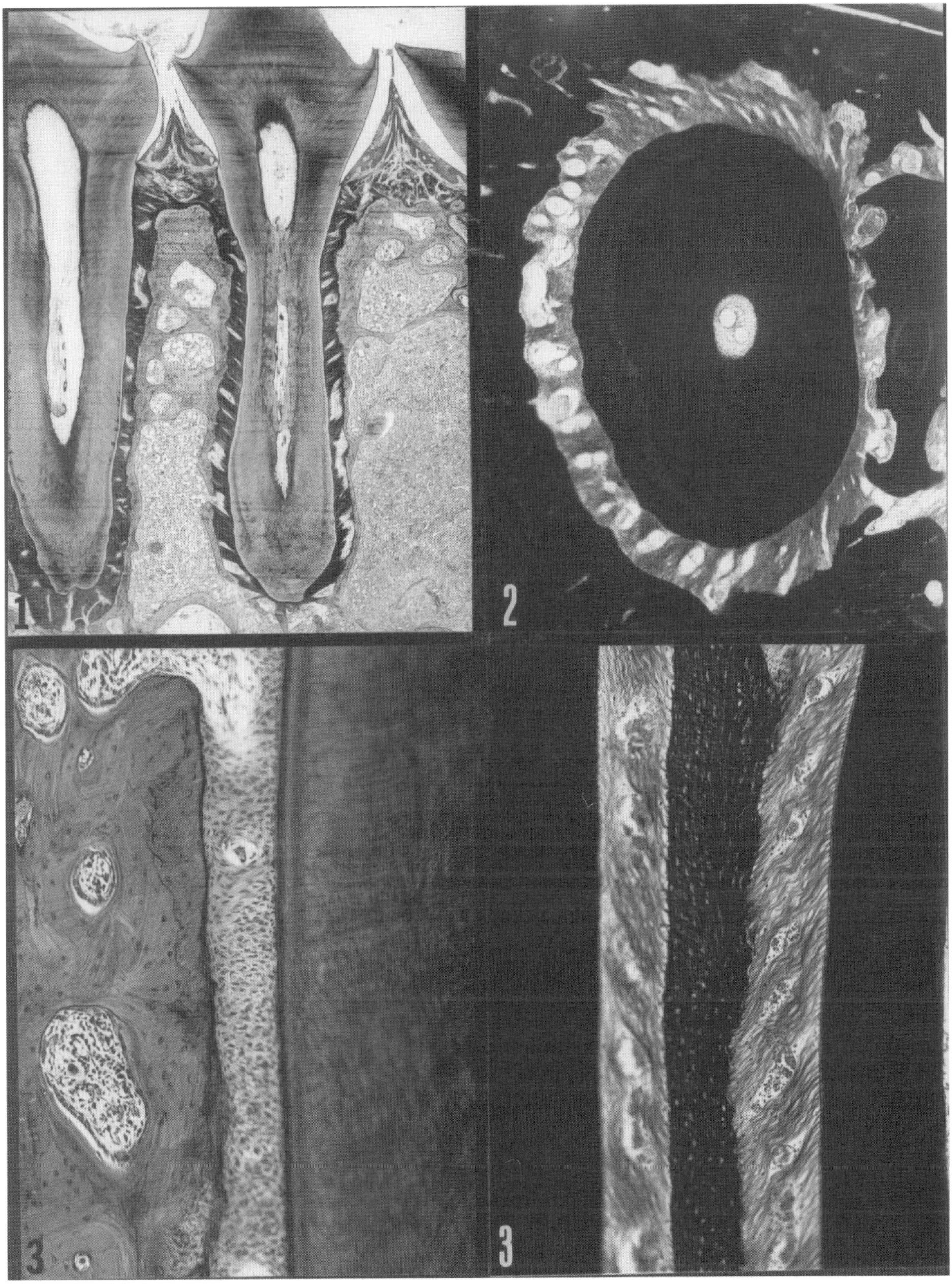

Plate 14-2

Fig. 14d. Mesio-distal section of adjacent premolar teeth. Note the organization of fiber groups of the PDL (Mallory's stain).

Fig. 14e. Cross section of premolar tooth below the level of the alveolar crest. Note circumferential fiber arrangement.

Fig. 14f. Note cellular structure of PDL.

Fig. 14g. Silver impregnated section of PDL illustrating the oblique fiber group.

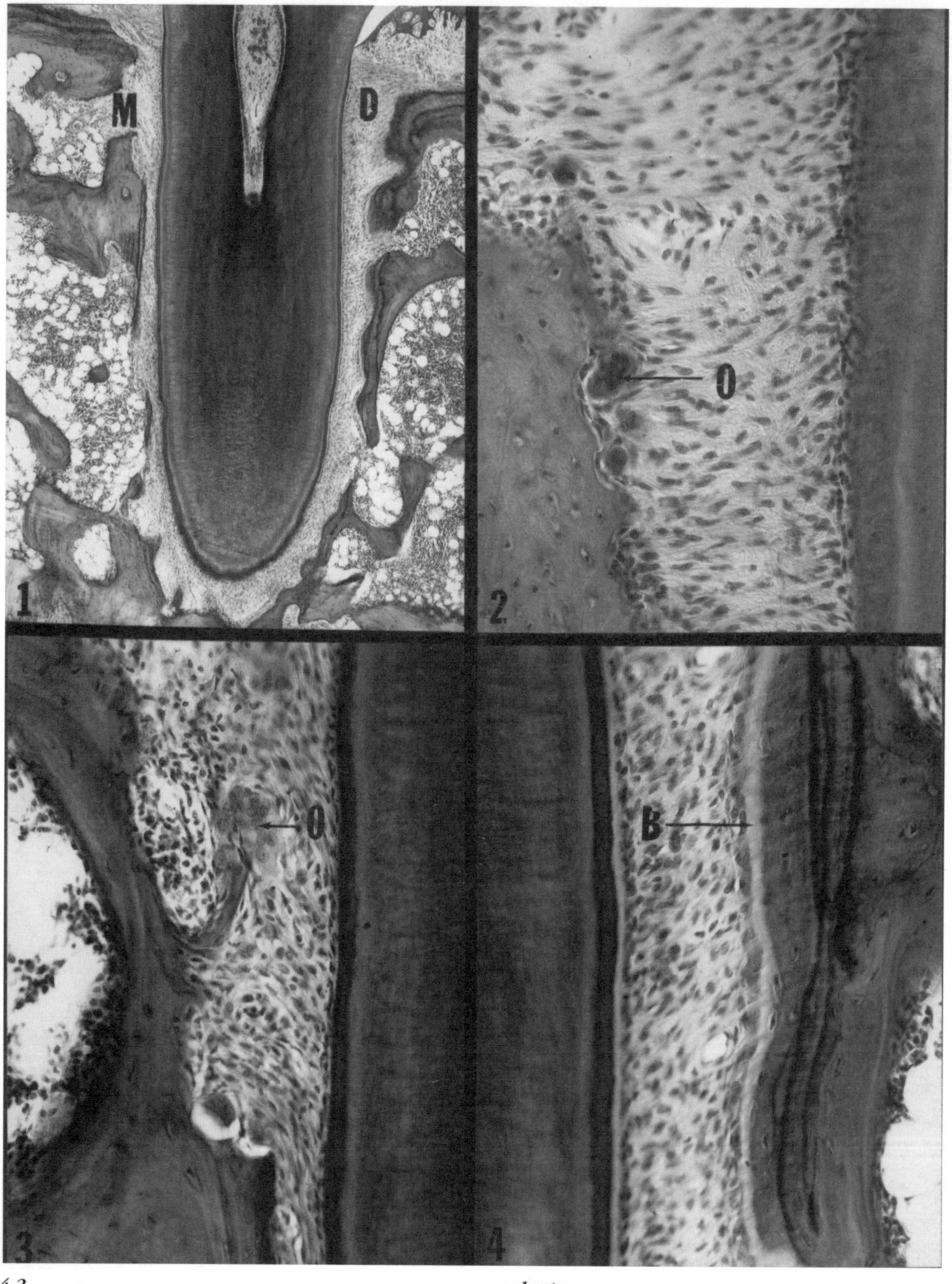

Plate 14-3

Fig. 14h. Section of upper premolar illustrating physiologic tooth movement. Compare the thickness of the PDL between the mesial and distal surfaces.

Fig. 14i. High magnification of alveolar crest region on mesial surface. Note presence of osteoclasts.

Fig. 14j. High magnification of midroot portion. Note osteoclasts.

Fig. 14k. High magnification of distal surface of midroot portion. Note presence of osteoid bone lining alveolar bone.

M-Mesial D-Distal O-Osteoclast B-Osteoid Bone

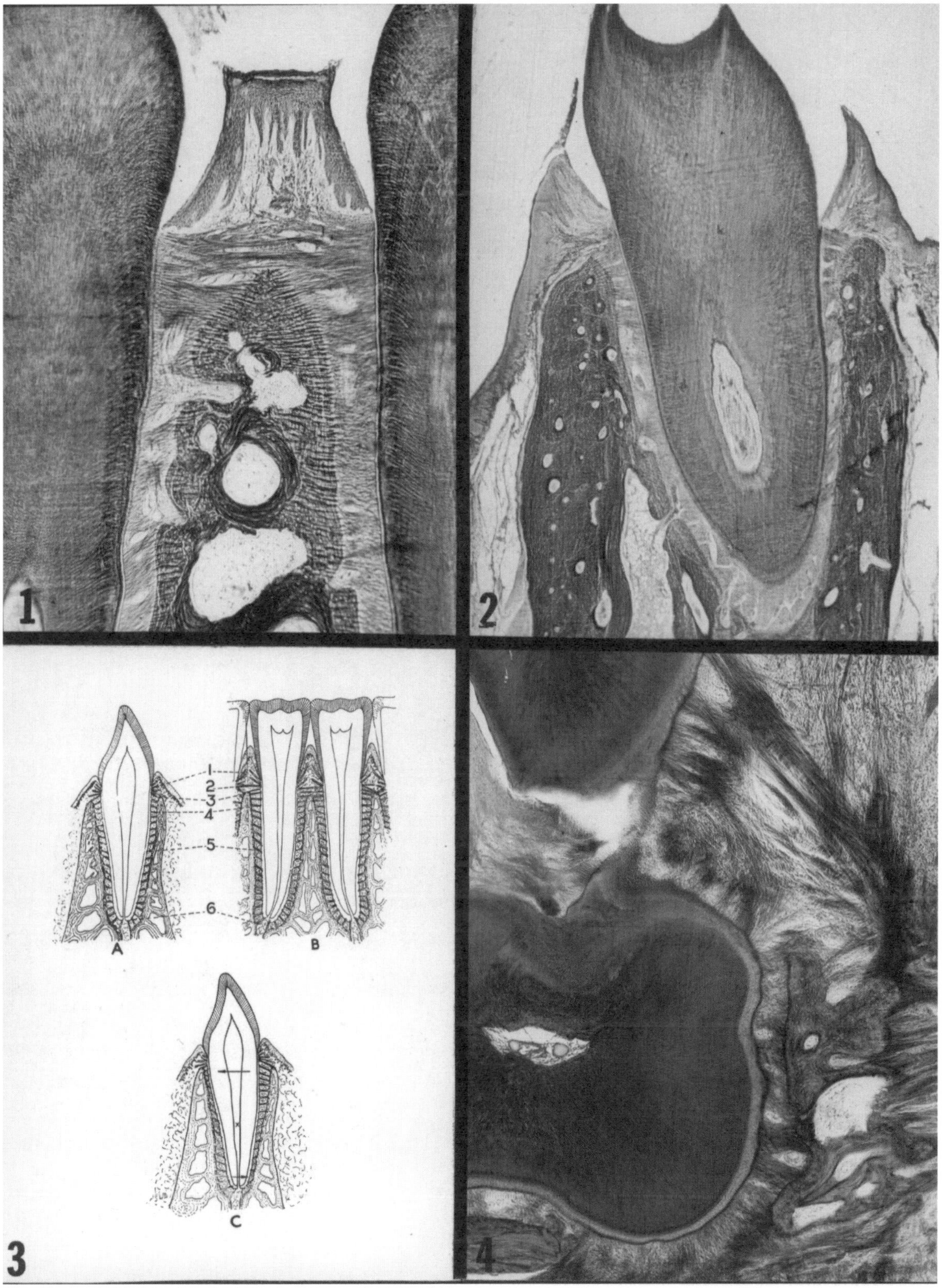

<u>Plate 14-4</u>

Fig. 14l. Silver impregnated section between upper molar and premolar. Note transeptal fibers, alveolar crest, horizontal and oblique fiber groups. Also observe the depth of Sharpey's fibers in the bone.

Fig. 14m. Silver stain, bucco-lingual section of lower molar. Note fiber arrangement.

Fig. 14n. Diagrammatic representation of fiber groups of PDL.

Fig. 14o. Ligamentum circulare located just above bony alveolar crest.

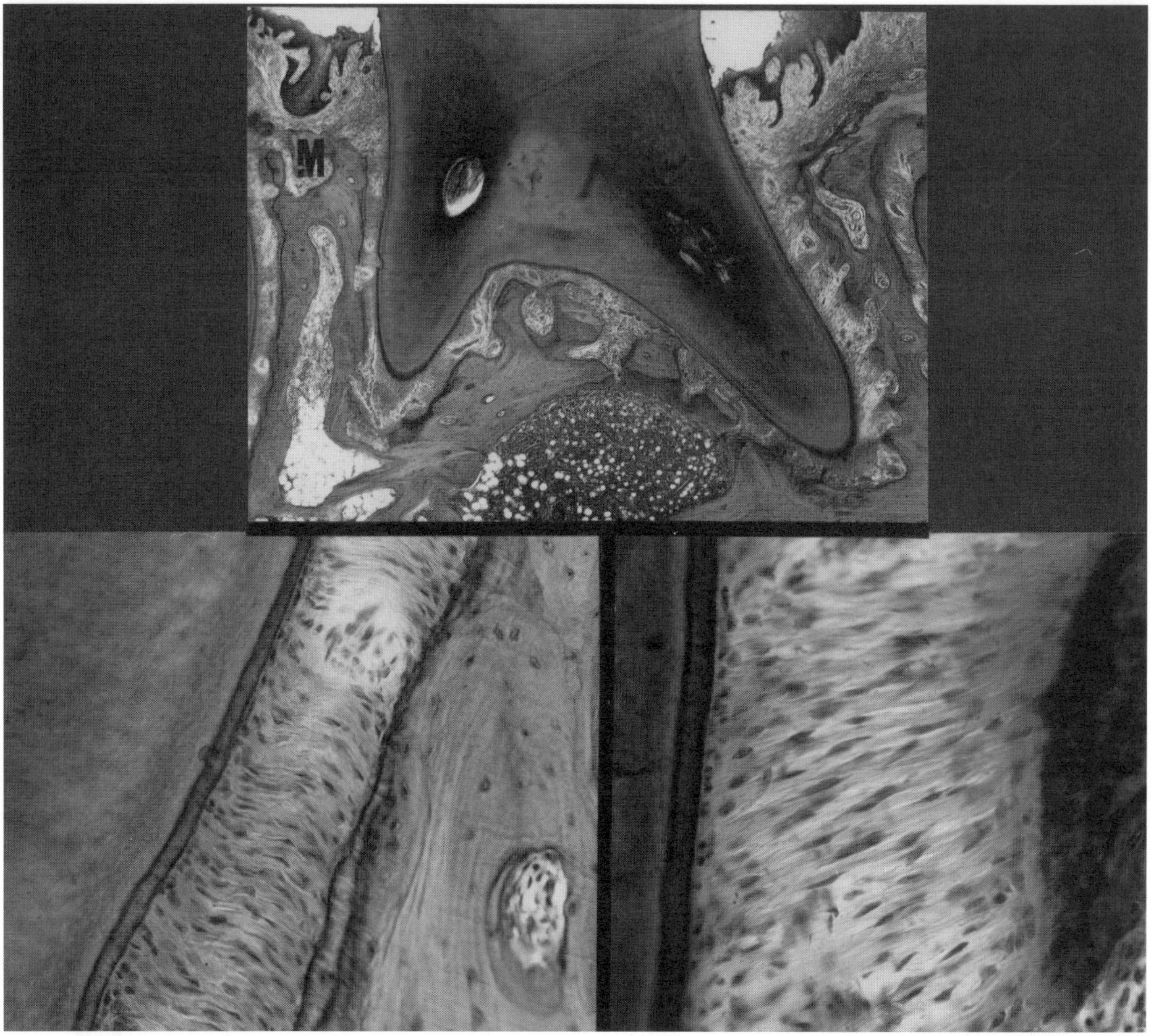

Plate 14-5

Fig. 14p. Mesio-distal section of a molar tooth that has had severe orthodontic pressures applied. Note stretching of fibers on side receiving pressure. Compression on opposite surface. Note severe compression on mesial surface of distal root.

Fig. 14q. Note narrowing of ligaments on the compression side with wavy fibers of OPDL.

Fig. 14r. Note tension and stretching of fibers. Note thinning of fibers in the midportion of the ligament space.

M-Mesial

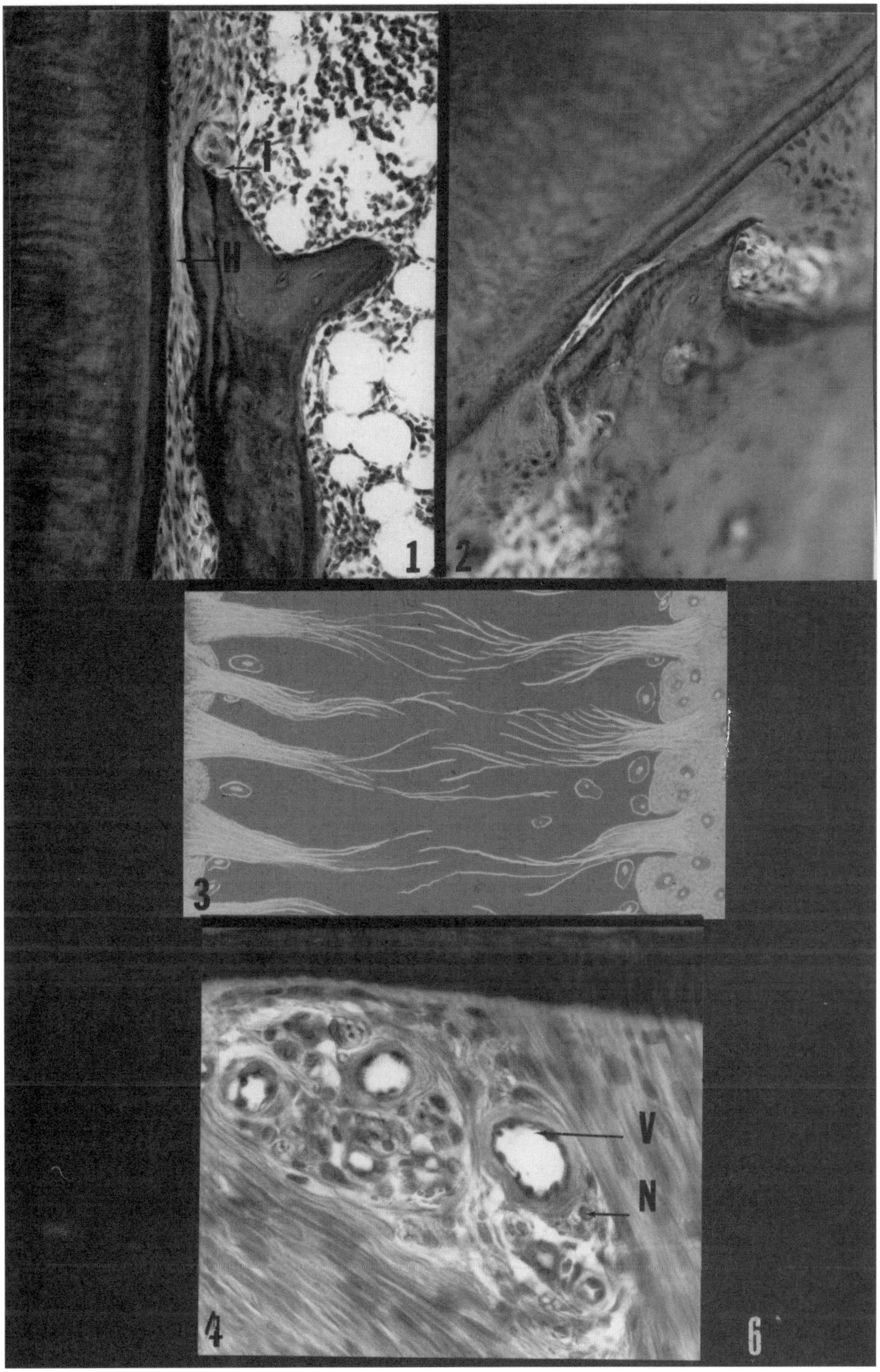

Plate 14-6

Fig. 14s. Note beginning hyalinization in a compression area. Observe internal resorption.

Fig. 14t. High magnification of severely compressed area following severe orthodontic pressure. Note hyalinization and destruction of PDL.

Fig. 14u. Diagram showing separation of PDL showing nerves and blood vessels between fiber bundles.

Fig. 14v.

H-Hyalinization V-Vessels N-Nerve

Editor's Note

Since the 1960s, findings of histological investigations of the periodontal ligament, particularly in humans, did not support the presence of the so-called "intermediate plexus." Further investigations since that time documented the functional role of fibroblasts not only in synthesizing and secreting collagenous fibers, but showed participation in their degradation as well. Thus the need for an intermediate plexus to accommodate periodontal fiber adaptation to tooth movement is negated by the action of fibroblasts.

Conceivably, periodontal fibroblasts can assemble collagen fibers into new attachments and contribute to removal of collagen fibers in old attachment sites. More recent investigations indicate a crucial role for the epithelial cell rests of Hertwig, which are present in the periodontal ligament in collagen degradation. These studies documented in vitro that these epithelial cells produce collagenase, an enzyme that specifically breaks down collagen fibers. In addition, these studies demonstrated that periodontal fibroblasts secrete an anti-collagenase factor.

These data support the notion of a controlled system to degrade collagen fibers to accommodate functional demands as well as force application to teeth as is the case in orthodontic therapy.

15.
Fractures

The voluntary muscle system evolved with the skeletal system and reflects its every demand. Just as the design and structure of a bone reflects the functional demands upon it, so do the location of its muscle attachments and the direction from which those muscles pull reflect the manner of their function. Neither the bones nor the muscles that control them can be considered independently, at least clinically. Nowhere is this more dramatically demonstrated than in the management of fractures of the jaws.

Fracture of Mandibular Corpus

The first case is taken directly from one of Moorehead's papers. A large, rugged young man of 23 years sustained a double fracture of the mandible from a blow in the jaw. One was an oblique fracture of the right condyle without apparent displacement and only revealed later by an x-ray of the entire head (Fig. 15a). The second was between the left canine and first bicuspid. The patient was hospitalized and immediate reduction by wiring was attempted. The patient stated that only three or four teeth were wired and that within 48 hours these were loose and the bite was open. Repeated cfforts failcd to close it and the patient was ulti mately dismissed.

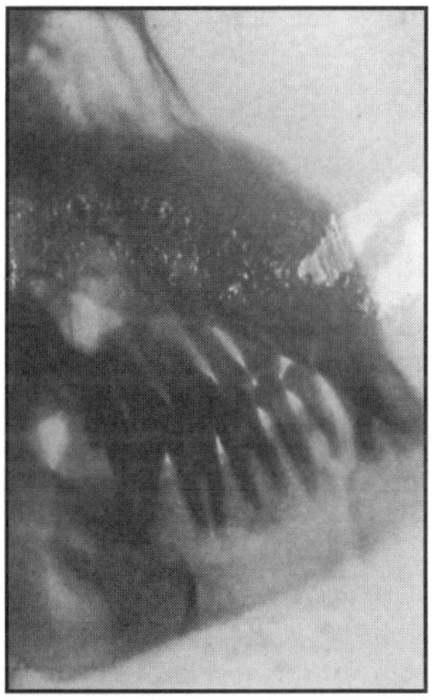

Fig. 15a. X-ray showing fracture between the left canine and the first premolar.

Seven months after the accident the patient sought consultation to see if anything further could be done for him. Plaster models of his condition at this time are shown in Fig. 15b. Only the premolars and molars on the left side were in occlusion and the x-ray revealed that there had been no union of the fracture. The patient complained of constant discomfort and was conscious of movement between the segments when he closed his jaws. There was a discharge of pus from around the neck of the premolar. The patient had fallen in weight from 175 pounds to 135 pounds, was living on a soft diet, and had become extremely despondent.

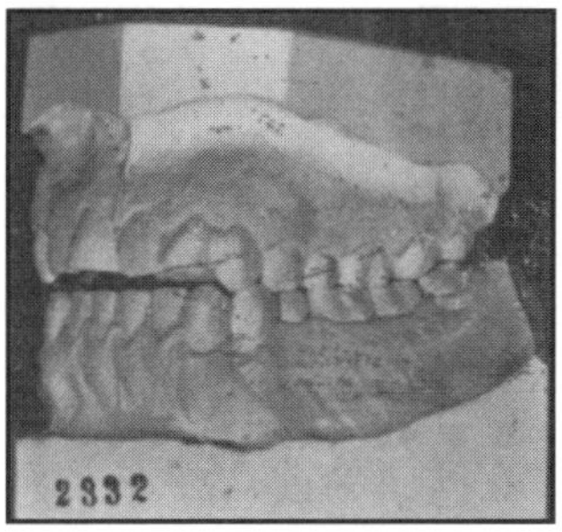

Fig. 15b. Plaster model showing displacement of anterior teeth.

In this case it was felt that an effort should be made to reduce the fracture properly before resorting to orthodontia. A full appliance was placed with bracket bands on all teeth as is shown in Fig. 15c. An upper arch bar (.022S x .028S) was used for anchorage. The lower arch bar was likewise made to fit the normal dental arch but was equipped with a spring loop at the site of the fracture. The arch itself was cut at this point, the loop permitting of some movement between the two segments when the arch was tied in. Only one small elastic was looped over the spurs at RAS and RBS for traction, and the case was dismissed for one week, the intention being to increase the traction at that time.

When the patient reported at the specified time, it was found that the ends of the arch segments in the loop now coincided, showing that the segments had once more been brought to their proper level. The change had occurred within 30 hours after the first appointment. The lower arch bar was replaced by a solid one to act as a splint. The occlusion was

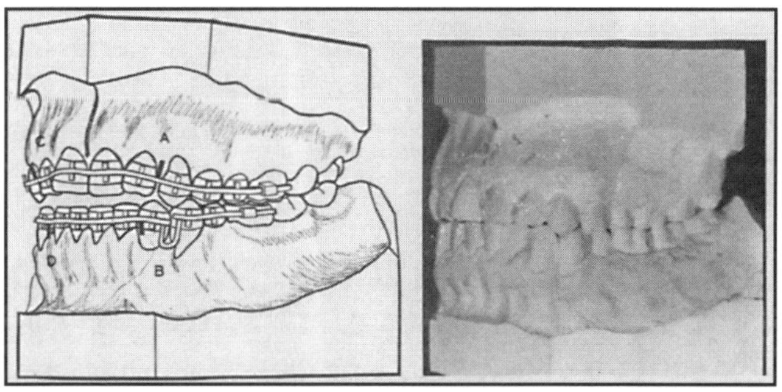

Fig. 15c. Left: Orthodontia mechanism in position. Right: Plaster model showing completion of treatment, with occlusion fully restored.

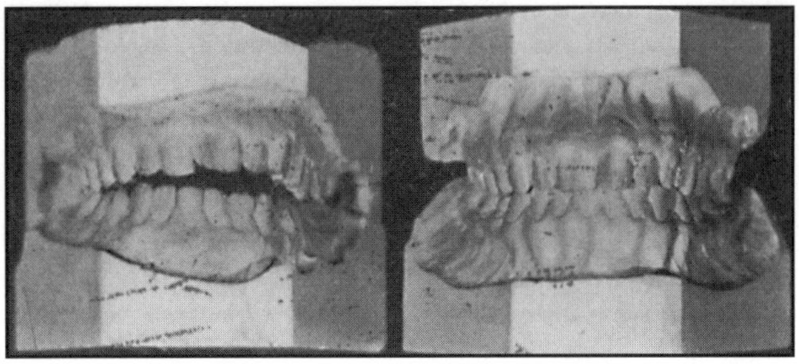

Fig. 15d. Left: Plaster model showing loss of occlusion. Right: Plaster model showing complete restoration of occlusion.

found to have improved considerably but was still slightly open in the incisor region. Traction was accordingly increased by the addition of an elastic between the spurs at RCS and RDS. The patient was now entirely comfortable, all discharge of pus had ceased at the bicuspid, and he was beginning to eat solid food (Fig. 15d).

Condyle Fracture (Case III)

Defying explanation on the basis of any factor other than restoration of the occlusion of the teeth to their preexisting relations are those cases which present fractures of the neck of the condyle. In these, the upward and forward rotation of the condyle always is accompanied by an anterior open bite which will not yield to closing by intermaxillary wiring. Another case taken from Moorehead's work illustrates this.

A girl, 17 years of age, was thrown through the windshield of an automobile in a head-on collision on August 8. She was hospitalized immediately. Examination revealed fractures of both condyloid processes of the mandible. Reduction by interdental wiring was undertaken two hours after the accident. Forty-eight hours after, it was discovered that the bite was open in front and numerous efforts to close it with wires failed. The case was dismissed seven weeks later.

When she was seen on October 5, x-rays revealed the position of the fragments. No movement could be demonstrated at the sites of the fractures. The bite was open 3/16 of an inch in the incisor region and only the second molars could be brought into contact. The patient could open and close her mouth but complained of discomfort, inability to chew her food and, most important, to the increase in the length of her face. Although more than seven weeks had elapsed since the accident, it was decided to attempt reduction by elastic traction. For this purpose, every tooth in both jaws was banded. There were two reasons for this. The length of treatment could not be predicted, and every precaution had to be taken against loosening teeth through overloading individual teeth. Furthermore, it had been decided that if union had already taken place, the patient would require a period of orthodontic management in order to restore the use of her masticatory apparatus.

After the appliance was placed, elastic bands were added between the upper and lower arches in the region of the canines. Only one small band was used at each site at first in order to avoid overloading the second molars, which would be the fulcrum. It was intended to increase the traction at the next appointment, one week later.

When the patient returned at the specified time, she stated that this result had been obtained within 18 hours after the elastics were inserted. She was entirely comfortable and was even eating comfortably. The elastics were continued for two months, when the entire appliance was removed.

One can only speculate on the forces that act to bring the fractured ends into correct apposition in these cases. It seems probable that the tensions set up by the displacement of the fragments into the dense fibrous tissues of the immediate environment are enough to accomplish it, if the masticatory musculature is maintained in the relaxed state.

As has been shown, the condyle in the intact bone is positioned superior-inferiorly by muscles running to the body of the mandible from above and below. Its anteroposterior position is determined by muscles running to the processes of the ramus from in front and in back. The external pterygoid muscle, originating on the lateral pterygoid lamina, runs backward and lateralward to the condyloid process, while the inferior horizontal fibers of the temporalis muscle run forward to the coronoid process. Thus, in fractures of the condyle neck, the coronoid process and the mandibular body to which it is attached cannot be drawn back while the condyle is displaced. The restraint offered by the capsular ligament causes this displacement by the external pterygoid to be a rotary movement, which carries the fractured neck in an upward, forward, and medialward direction.

Inaccessibility makes these fractures difficult to manage, and numerous methods have been employed for their reduction. The most obvious is the direct surgical approach followed by manual manipulation and wiring of the fragments. This frequently has unfortunate sequellae such as the tearing of the capsule, bleeding followed by scar tissue formation, and limitation of movement. These risks have made this method increasingly unpopular.

At the other extreme is the total avoidance of interference, which is frequently the preferred course with the young patient. Even in the face of considerable displacement, remodeling and restoration of normal function seems to proceed rapidly following a period of two or three weeks rest with the teeth wired, provided that the previous state of the occlusion has been exactly restored. It will be recognized by the reader that the fracture has left the tension of the temporalis muscle unopposed, and that the mandible may be somewhat retracted on this side. The degree of such retraction can be judged by the orthodontist from the occlusion, and if it is excessive it can be corrected in the later stages of management by applying light elastic traction from the upper canine region to the lower molar area. This also will act to unlock any impaction of the fractured ends and hasten reunion.

Knowledge of what may be expected following efforts at reduction of subcondylar fractures is woefully incomplete and rests largely on clinical evidence. Such evidence does not parallel findings gained from animal experimentations, as for example in the rat, the pig, and the monkey, where total extirpation of the condyle has been followed by complete regeneration with only slight effect on the attainment of complete growth of the mandible. Indeed, in the case of one pig, the growth of the ramus and condyle on the operated side exceeded that of the other side.

The author inclines to the belief that the marked difference between the animal and the human in this regard results from the profound adaptations that have accompanied and made possible the attainment of the erect posture. As has been pointed out earlier, the reorientation of the body necessitated the enlistment of the muscles of mastication as part of the postural chain. The substitution of the external pterygoid for gravity in mouth opening assured the patentcy of the airway during this act while simultaneously concentrating the most anterior of the postural gravitational forces in the chin area.

Frederick B. Moorehead states: "We have cited these cases to emphasize first the value of traction in reducing a fracture which cannot be reduced by any other method except an open operation, which should never be employed except possibly in edentulous jaws with marked displacement; and second, to call attention to the necessity of using orthodontic appliances and the cooperation of a trained orthodontist or a dentist familiar with orthodontic methods in case a specialist is not available. While all fractures belong naturally in the province of the surgeon, he cannot manage old fractures of the jaw with the same skill as the orthodontist. This is a splendid place for teamwork. The skills of both are needed. The wise surgeon will ask for the services of the orthodontist and the wise orthodontist will ask for the services of the surgeon. It is rather too bad when anyone transgresses the field of practice which belongs to another by virtue of specific training and experience."

Principles of Management of Fractures of the Jaws

The voluntary muscle system evolved with the skeletal system and reflects its every demand. Just as the design and structure of a bone reflects the functional demands upon it, so do the location of its muscle attachments and the direction from which those muscles pull reflect the manner of their function. Neither the bones nor the muscles that control them can be considered independently, at least clinically. Nowhere is this more dramatically demonstrated than in the management of fractures of the jaws.

Muscle Behavior in Facial Fractures

Muscles are constantly under tension, and they will immediately shorten if given the opportunity to do so. Thus, these ideas on muscle function can be confirmed by the behavior of bone fragments following fracture. There are a number of areas of muscle attachment on the mandible, and the stresses operating on them are in different directions (Fig. 15e). At the condyle neck there is the forward and medial pull exerted by the external pterygoid

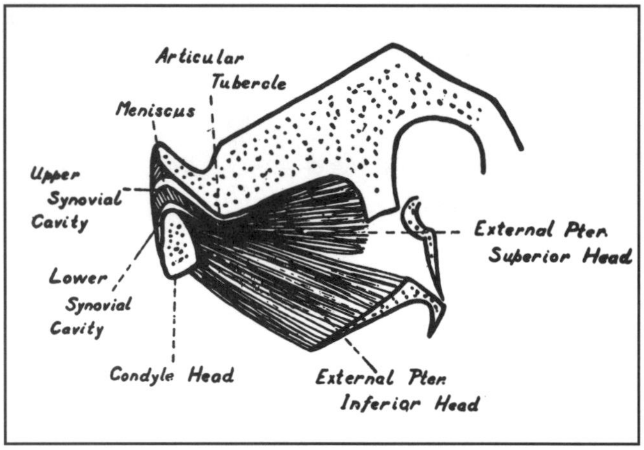

Fig. 15e.

muscle, while on the coronoid process there is upward and backward force operating from the temporalis. The rest of the ramus is under the influence of the masseter and internal pterygoid, their mean pull being in an upward and forward direction. Anteriorly, the suprahyoid muscles exert a downward and backward pull (Fig. 15f).

In a unilateral fracture of the condyle neck, the condyle is rotated forward, medially, and upward by the pull of the external pterygoid and the ramus moves slightly backward because of the unopposed pull on the coronoid process from the temporalis. Aside from this latter change, little other alteration is apparent in the position of the mandible until the mouth is opened. Then the external pterygoid on the uninjured side brings that condyle forward without a similar movement taking place on the injured side, and the jaw is seen to swing toward the side of the fracture.

Fractures of the coronoid process are rare. They would be expected to retract the process alone upward and backward into the temporal fossa. Fractures at the junction of the body and ramus result in an upward and forward rotation of the ramus induced by the pull of the masseter and internal pterygoid, while the body tends to be drawn down by the tensions from the suprahyoid group, especially the mylohyoid.

The degree of displacement of the fragments in bilateral fractures of the body of the mandible depends on the force and direction of the original blow as well as on the muscle tensions operating afterward, and both may be modified by impaction at the sites of the fractures. If the fragments do not impact and the fractures are toward the front of the mandible (lateral canine areas), there is danger of choking. The hyoid bone, which is the foundation for the tongue, as well as the tongue itself, both are suspended in front from the genial tubercles on the internal surface of the symphysis. With the release of their tension, the entire tongue is drawn downward and backward, occluding the airway.

Traditionally, fractures of bone have been managed by immobilizing the parts with some form of support such as a splint, or by holding them together with wires, staples, and screws. In all cases, the objective has been the prevention of any movement that might disturb the healing process at the break. Perfect apposition is rarely possible owing to existing muscle forces and inaccessibility, but failure to attain it has not been considered serious because experience has shown that the preexisting bone form is restored in time by deposition and resorption of bone, i.e. remodeling.

It would be expected that in the treatment of

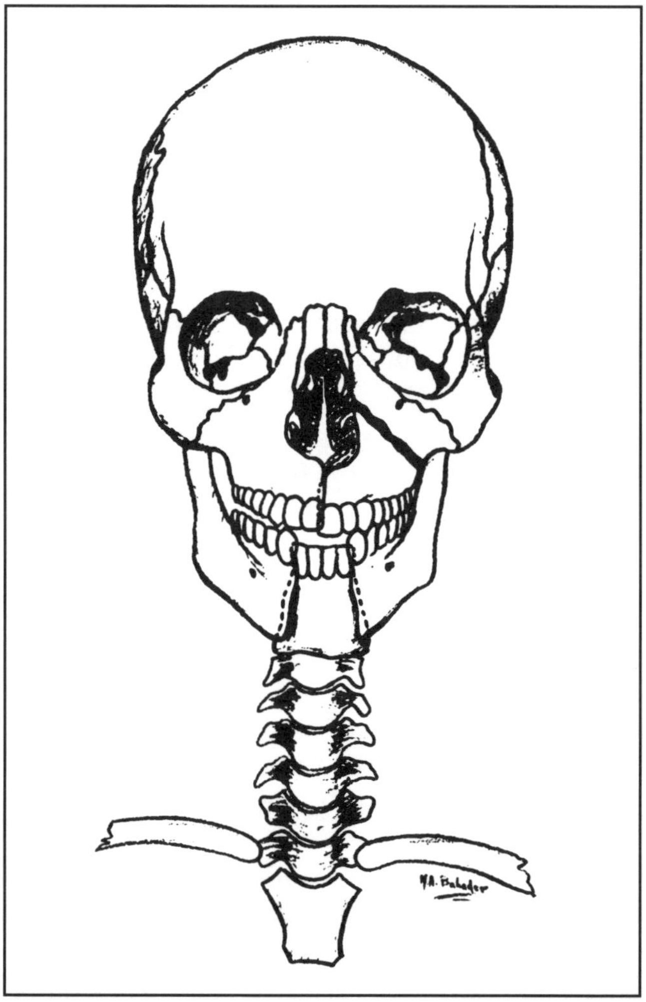

Fig. 15f.

jaw fractures the same tenets would be relied on as those that have governed fracture reductions in general, namely, firm fixation and immobilization. The presence of teeth offers not only ready accessibility but an admirable means of attachment, and direct interdental wiring has long been a favored technique. In spite of these obvious advantages, fractures of the jaws pose problems more critical than in most other parts of the skeleton. Esthetics is more important in the face than almost anywhere else in the body, and incorrectly set fractures can be extremely disfiguring. Furthermore, the disfigurement diminishes more slowly than in areas where function is heavier and more constant. Almost perfect approximation of the fragments must be attained if preexisting occlusal relaxations are to be restored. Failure in this can lead to traumatizing of teeth and joints. Beyond this the immobilization of the jaws through wiring of teeth inhibits mastication throughout the entire period of healing and adjustment.

The most important requirement is the understanding of the intimate bone-muscle-function relation that must dictate the reduction of the fractures of the face. I was introduced to this concept by watching and occasionally helping Frederick B. Moorehead, professor of maxillofacial surgery, at the University of Illinois, who I believe originated it. From him I learned that even the strongest muscle can be fatigued by any unremitting force, even gravity or the pull of the smallest or weakest elastic band; how the same muscle, given even slight opportunity to rest, could reestablish its resting length even to the stretching of wires that had been employed to hold the teeth together. I also came to appreciate more fully the close harmony that exists between the occlusal pattern of an individual and the muscles that control his jaw movements. Finally, it was evident that if occlusion could be restored exactly to its original state without the orthodontic movement of individual teeth, the bone fragments that held them would of necessity be in their correct relations to each other. A few cases will illustrate these points.

Management of Maxillary Fractures

The maxilla has no muscles running to it from other parts that can influence its position in space. Hence, there are no muscle tensions to displace the fragments following fracture. Displacements of the total maxilla or any of its parts reflect only the magnitude and direction of the injuring force. But here again, the objective is the reestablishment of the preexisting occlusion.

In simple fractures involving only the alveolar process, it is sufficient to align the teeth with the fingers and apply a small section of arch wire to splint them to adjacent sound teeth. If only one maxilla, that is, one half of the upper jaw is fractured, it may be controlled by banding in the displaced segment, together with the mandibular teeth, applying a small arch wire to each part. Subsequent connecting of these two wires with elastics will usually be all that is necessary to reduce the fracture and restore the occlusion.

The great increase in the number of automobile accidents in which passengers sustain heavy blows on the middle face from directly in front has led to an increasing number of cases in which the two maxillae are detached from their cranial support.

Mandibular fractures are a frequent accompaniment. These must be managed first because the spatial position of the mandible is determined by muscles and furnishes the operator a dependable guide for the correct functional position of the maxillary fragments.

A moment's reflection on the anatomy involved in this type of accident is enough to reveal its seriousness. The maxilla is attached to its foundation, the brain case, at only three points: (1) at its junction with the outer table of the frontal bone near the midline, (2) at its junction with the zygomatic bone at the side, and (3) at its junction with the pterygoid process of the sphenoid bone in back. These are the stress-ways which carry functional loads from the maxilla. Of these three stress-ways, the first two are part of the external shield of compact bone covering the internal face. It can immediately be realized that if the maxilla or maxillae have been displaced to any extent, all three of the supporting stress-ways must have suffered fracture. What of the structures behind that external shield?

All of the bones of the internal upper face are extremely light and delicate, acting for the most part merely as partitions between different functional systems. At the midline is the nasal septum, hardly a sturdy structure. The lateral wall of the nose above the level of the orbital floor acts only as a thin cover for the ethmoidal air cells, and below this level helps to close the maxillary sinus. The lateral wall is extended in back by the perpendicular plate of the palatine bone and the medial pterygoid lamina, both also very thin bones. The orbit is separated from the ethmoidal air cells only by the lamina papyracea, whose name betrays its delicacy. The superior and inferior orbital fissures form the posterior and most of the lateral boundaries of the orbit. Thus, there is no sturdy articulation except that at the zygomaticofrontal junction, which is one of the major stress pathways. Some idea of the widespread derangement of the nasal cavity, the ethmoidal and maxillary sinuses, and occasionally even the orbits following displacement of the maxillae, can be realized from this.

How can fractures of such a number of delicate bone partitions be reduced with any certainty that they will be as they were previously? Since there are no muscles attached to the maxillae that can displace them by shortening, these bones can be restored to their correct positions largely by manual manipulation. The best guide to the correct position is the occlusion of the teeth as it existed prior to injury. In many cases, this is all that is necessary, as shown by the following case.

A young man fell asleep at the wheel of his automobile and crashed into a light pole. Both maxillae were crushed lingually within the lower arch. His dentist examined him and referred him to an orthodontist, no oral surgeon being available at the time. Intraoral examination revealed an upper cast, gold partial denture carrying several anterior teeth. Questioning revealed that it was new and had been uncomfortable and the patient had removed it some time prior to the accident. Embarrassed by his lack of front teeth in a public conveyance he had managed to reinsert the denture and seat it before arriving at the orthodontist's office. He had reduced his own fractures and required no further treatment.

Another case which illustrates even better the close interdependence of the occlusion of the teeth and the associated skeleton of the face was that of a truck driver, who had been involved in a head-on collision. He sustained a complete horizontal fracture with posterior displacement of the maxillae. Sides of the upper dental arch were in lingual crossbite but were in contact with the lower only at the last molars. There was an anterior open bite of nearly three-quarters of an inch, with a downward and backward thrust of the upper jaw. There had been extensive damage to the ethmoidal labyrinth, and bleeding into the throat was extensive. After three days in the hospital, when hemorrhage was controlled and the danger of infection seemed over, the patient was referred to a local orthodontist whose success in the treatment of such extensive fractures was known locally. The orthodontist seated him in the dental chair and faced him sitting on a stool. Digital manipulation was sufficient to move the two maxillae laterally until they were approximately above their usual occlusal positions. The dental chair was then rotated and its back dropped so that the patient's head was resting in the orthodontist's lap. Making a sling of his laced fingers and hands, he then exerted sudden and sufficient force on the lower border of the mandible to bring the teeth into occlusion. He dismissed the patient with instructions to bite hard on his teeth at frequent intervals, as in the Rogers biting exercises. Within 24 hours the teeth were settled into their previous positions and all his discomfort had subsided.

This type of treatment is in marked contrast to that usually employed when efforts are made to completely immobilize the parts. Complete immobilization is rarely attainable, and indeed there are those who maintain that a slight degree of movement is desirable and actually promotes healing. Furthermore, considering the very delicate partitions which must be brought into approximation if the preexisting anatomical relations are to be restored, it would seem apparent that only by the sheerest accident could this be obtained by the immobilization of the parts either through splinting or the formerly common practice of forming a plaster cast for the head with an outer bow around the face, to which wires from various intraoral appliances can be attached only by piercing the cheeks.

Reading list:

Moorehead, Frederick B., and Dewey, Kaethe W. *Pathology of the Mouth.* Philadelphia: W.B. Saunders, 1925.

16.
Repair and Adjustment

It requires but a moment of reflection to realize that living things could exist only fleetingly were they not endowed with means for repairing themselves or of making adjustment to damaging vicissitudes of their existence. These protective measures evolved simultaneously with the tissues, organs, and systems which they were adapted to guard. Each tissue has its own distinct reactionary response.

Epithelium

Excluding gravity, the environmental factors to which living forms have adapted have been those that acted principally on their surfaces. During the earliest stages, ectoderm covered the entire outside of the body and its involutions were such that it came to line those cavities which are the principal concern of the dentist, namely the mouth and gut. Thus the lining and the covering must be thought of as outer surfaces at which the environment comes in direct physical contact with the body. The external covering is called epithelium.

Epithelium exhibits a wide range of adaptations to a myriad of environmental factors. For present purposes, consideration will be limited to only those that might be thought of as repair or replacement processes: its responses to the wear of function. This varies quantitatively as the degree of function varies, although the response is in kind under a variety of conditions.

Epithelium is the squamous cell covering of mesenchymal tissue; the mesenchyme usually being papillated. New epithelial cells form constantly at the junction and move toward the surface, their nucleii becoming kyphotic in the process and dissapearing entirely from the cells of the surface layers. It is at the free surface that the unique adaptive capacities of epithelium are most evident.

Under ordinary conditions of function, the surface nucleii-free cells are sloughed off at a rate that matches the proliferation of new cells at the basement membrane. The rate of turnover varies with the degree of function, the palmar surfaces of the hands and feet being high compared to those surfaces not subject to wide extremes of temperature, as everyone is aware.

Mesenchyme

Mesenchyme is the parent tissue of blood, connective tissue, cartilage, and bone and the results of many of its responses can be seen and measured. Its basic cellular phases are not within the scope of this book. These are treated in detail by Maximow and reviewed by Schour; they should be studied there.

A broken bone would render an animal helpless were it not for the repair process, but there are other properties in bone that are not so apparent. Bones have evolved to serve a number of functions which range from that of withstanding great shocks and weights to that of acting as a framework for delicate membranes. Microscopically, the bone tissue involved in these two functions is identical, but a substitution of one for the other would be impossible because of their differing phylogenetic derivations. Each bone of the body of each species has been gradually adapted in accordance with functional demands until at present it seems to reflect perfectly the harmony between form and function. This applies not only to its gross form but also to the trabeculae and the course and number of its Haversian systems. From all of this emerges a law of bone design: A normal bone represents the least amount of material, most efficiently arranged to carry the peak load of its several functions.

As stated before, the architecture, external form, and internal arrangement of trabeculae is an inherited pattern, and this pattern is a diagram of forces that oppose stresses the particular bone has been evolved to resist. Ordinarily bones would carry much heavier loads than are normally put upon them, as witness the man or woman who gains 80 or 90 pounds over a period of years without any bowing of the legs. This would be a normal stimulus since the increased load would be directed along the lines that the bone was phylogenetically designed to withstand.

On the other hand, if a very light force acts upon a bone in a direction in which it was not phylogenetically designed to withstand, deformity results. In this connection, one might cite the cowboy whose legs become bowed through the lateral pressure of only their own weight against a horse, a fraction of the load they withstand in their normal direction. And a more pertinent example is that where the masticatory load is greatly increased. Primitive man developed biting power up to 300 pounds per square inch without deformity, yet a tiny inflated rubber sack in the vestibule of the mouth will cause measurable narrowing of the dental arches in 48 hours. The first would be a normal, the second an abnormal, stimulus.

In addition to the direction of the force is the matter of the type of force employed. Most natural, functional forces are intermittent, and this permits rest. No tissue can work continuously without time for repairing itself, and bone is no exception. If force is applied in the same direction against two bones, one steadily and one intermittently, the bone subjected to the steady force will give way much more rapidly than the other.

The most remarkable characteristic of bone, however, is the nature of its response to any force. When pressure is brought to bear against inanimate things they tend to give way before the force; bone on the other hand may be forced to yield to the point where its form may be changed, but microscopic examination will reveal that its internal trabecular arrangement has been altered to better resist the new force. In short, bone builds against stress.

From these facts it should be apparent that before trying to apply treatment to any bone, it would be helpful to know something of its phylogenetic development as well as a good deal about the normal functional forces it was called upon to withstand. A very good example of this has been demonstrated in experimental work on animal dentures.

In selecting two animal species of different habits, such as carnivora and herbivora, it has been found that depression movements are quite easily accomplished in the first, but buccal or lingual movements are very difficult. The teeth of the herbivora react exactly opposite, yielding easily to expansion or contraction but not at all to depression. In other words, each reveals the direction in which it was phylogenetically designed to withstand stress, but yields when force is applied in a different direction. Thus the reactive capacity of the bone is shown to be "species linked."

In the law of bone design there is a hidden implication that also must be remembered. The phrase "least amount of material" actually means that this amount is all that is necessary if all accessory factors of resistance are present. It has been seen how the bones of the calvaria differ in their structure depending on whether or not additional protection-is provided by musculature. In a similar manner, bones that are aided by other structures are not as robust as they would have to be if they were required to withstand force alone. There is no better place to study this arrangement than in the bones that support the teeth, namely the maxilla and mandible.

The maxilla is a bone of many functions, and each function places different demands upon it. Its role as an "air conditioner" requires that enormous free surface of delicate structure be compressed into a small area in exactly the same manner as that found in the radiator of an automobile. Yet this same bone is called upon to withstand some of the greatest stress borne by the body, namely mastication.

We have seen in the study of anatomy how all of the masticatory stresses are carried by the outer shell of bone and quickly transmitted across space to areas of the head capable of absorbing them. What has not been seen thus far is that every other factor which enters into the organ of mastication is so designed as to permit this bone to be more efficient in its several roles. These accessory factors make definite supportive contributions to the maintenance of a condition of balance within the denture. Most malocclusions of environmental etiology in man seem to arise through the failure of one or more of these factors to play its correct part or to make more or less than its normal contribution to balance. In the past, these various factors have been referred to as "forces of occlusion."

Teeth must be looked upon as appendages of the body and not as an integral part of it. They have no power of self-adjustment or repair once they are formed, aside from the formation of secondary dentin. On the other hand, their functional efficiency depends upon the very precise relationships among the teeth of the individual jaws as well as between those of the two jaws. Since their function causes wear and since wear usually decreases eficiency, some means of adjustment is invariably found to be present.

A study of lower animal forms reveals a number of such provisions, each related to the level of evolutionary development. Thus the lowest tooth-bearing form, the fishes, rely on a perpetual sucession of teeth; if one is torn out, another is formed in its place. At this phylogenetic level, the teeth are simple cones and are used only for prehension. Perpetual succession has continued to the present day in the fish and the reptile and is combined with other types of adjustment in the buccal teeth of the elephant, the kangaroo, and the manatee. In these forms the teeth move forward through the jaws as they are worn out and are shed at the diastema at the corner of the mouth.

Perpetual growth is a type of adjustment present where the use of the tooth results in great wear. In these forms, enamel dentin and cementum are constantly being added at the proximal ends while the distal end is being worn. The rodent incisor is the first example that springs to mind, but the tusks of elephants, walruses, and boars also are teeth of perpetual growth. All must be looked upon as prehensile in function, that is, they permit the animal to get at his food.

In animals in which the diet requires a fine trituration of food, e.g., the breaking and tearing of starch granules as by the grazers and ruminants, a mechanism of perpetual eruption is found. The teeth, although fully formed early in life, erupt continually. Thus, they adjust to the marked wear of their occlusal surfaces. In these forms there is an additional factor which is combined with eruption in the interest of maintaining efficiency. This is the design of the tooth itself. In the horse or steer, the grinding teeth of the buccal segments present an unbroken occlusal surface from front to back and the teeth lean against each other; those in front lean backward, and those in the back lean forward. Interproximal wear is thus taken up, and the contacting surfaces are kept tight by eruption.

Tooth Drift

Mesial drift has long been a favored term of the orthodontist to explain those malocclusions which present partially or completely blocked out bicuspid teeth or a forward leaning of canine teeth with crowded incisors. This reflects a belief that occlusal force on the molars, which appear to stand mesially inclined, contributes a foward vector through the contact points which leads to a break in the arch at the canine-lateral junction.

A moment's thought would reveal that an identical condition would result from other causes, e.g., eruption of the permanent canines before the jaws (particularly the apical base) had expanded sufficiently to accommodate it, or any unbalanced buccal force such as tense musculature operating in the canine area before the arch was complete. It must be kept in mind that the apices of the teeth are their most stable points and that most tooth movements, aside from those accompanying mastication, are of a tipping nature with the apices acting as their centers.

Investigations are revealing that these quite obvious factors serve only to modify a more fundamental mechanism of adjustment. Every species has its own peculiar combination of attributes to enable it to procure and prepare its own particular diet most efficiently and to maintain that efficiency through less obvious adaptations. In flesh eaters the heavy mediolateral forces operating on the carnasial and canine teeth, which would be expected to drive the uppers buccally and the lowers lingually, actually witness lingual drift of the upper teeth and the buccal drift of the lower. This was shown experimentally by grinding the contacting surfaces of the teeth of cats to simulate more than average wear. Avital dye (lead acetate) was injected to make visible the nature and pattern of bone reactions in the alveolar process. Low-power microscopic examination revealed deposition on the surfaces facing in the direction from which the forces were coming and resorption on the opposite sides, indicating a drift against force. Similar studies on other species of animals have revealed different drift tendencies of various groups of teeth, which serve demands in addition to that of maintaining contact relations. In rodents, the molar segment drifts distally in spite of a marked mesial inclination of the teeth. In swine, a posterior and buccal movement of the premolars and molars accompanies the development of the long snout. This behavior is common to many animals serving to keep the chief chewing teeth in a relation of maximum mechanical advantage relative to the muscles of mastication.

The behavior of the incisors in most animals except flesh eaters and those living on aquatic plants (hippopotami) exhibit strong drift toward the midline, which is probably attributable both to their mesial inclination and their inherent drift tendencies. In rodents, it is markedly accentuated by the lifelong growth of these teeth.

It is not possible to draw conclusions regarding drift of human teeth with the assurance one has in animal studies because the same type of evidence, namely, vital staining and histologic tissue sectioning, is not available.

The incisors, however, offer unmistakable evidence of a mesial drift tendency in the clinical procedure of palate splitting. The forceful midline separation of the maxillae is followed by a reestablishment of interproximal contact between the central incisors in the space of a month or so. Both of these would seem to implicate the periodontal ligament rather than the tooth. The canines and the buccal teeth offer no such irrefutable evidence of their normal drift tendencies in spite of the frequent claims that they are in a forward direction. Points of reference outside of the denture are unreliable, because they too are being moved continually by remodelling.

The chief interest of the orthodontist is the drift of teeth centered around their influence on the etiology of malocclusion and the effect of tooth loss on the remaining teeth. A study was made by Seward, in 1965, on the results of the extraction of deciduous molars. It was based on findings derived from serial models and cephalometric x-rays. He summarized his findings as follows:

"In the maxilla all extraction spaces closed. All save one closed by mesial migration of the teeth distal to the extraction space. Space loss ranged from 2.0 to 7.3 mm. In the mandible all except two extraction spaces closed. All space losses greater than 2.0 mm. were brought about mainly by a distal movement of the teeth mesial to the space."

At present, the most scientifically satisfactory evidence of drift is that to be derived from the vital staining of animals. This indicates that certain nonfunctional drift movements occur in the same direction as that in which the bone which holds them is growing. Thus in the pig mandible, the growth pattern of which is strikingly similar to that of the human, the buccal teeth drift posterolaterally as the mandible does likewise. In humans, a continuation of such movement beyond maturity could help to explain the "falling in" of the mouth in senility. Thus, it would seem that all tooth movements are not due to obvious environmental mechanical forces.

Teeth as Tools

Man is the only animal having a denture unbroken by a diastema (and therefore cannot enjoy the protection it affords), and must rely on tooth design for such protection. This is thought to play an important role in maintaining the efficiency of his denture. Teeth are cutting tools in the strictest sense of the word, and a very striking analogy may be drawn between these organs and the tools fashioned by humans.

The vital part of any tool is that part which is presented to the work to be done. This is nothing more nor less than a thin edge, or even a point. All the rest of the tool is for the purpose of making the edge effective. Of recent date, we have witnessed the introduction of a tool that consists of only an edge and nothing more—the butter or cheese cutter employed by the grocer. For the most part, however, tools need more than an edge because of the work they must do and the material they must work upon.

The edge of a cutting tool must possess the quality of hardness if it is to work efficiently over long periods of time. Thus, man fashions his tools out of alloys capable of taking a high degree of temper (tool steel) or tips his drill point with diamond. In a like manner and serving an identical purpose, the teeth are covered on their coronal portions with the hardest substance found in the animal kingdom: enamel.

Very hard substances do not possess at the same time another quality that is necessary if the usage is heavy. This is toughness. Thus, that portion of the tool which supports the brittle cutting edge is composed of a materal which gives strength sufficient to permit the application of force to do the work without breaking. Again in teeth there is a parallel situation, with the tough dentin acting to give sufficient strength to support the enamel.

A tool as such is valueless; it must be powered and driven, and for this to be accomplished it must be grasped. Thus tools have handles with a great variety in design. Well-designed tools adhere to certain principles. The handles are of a size that permits a good grasp, but in most cases no more, unless balance demands it. There is no need to supply surface that will not be used. Handles are also of a shape that is best adapted for the particular hand grasp to be employed and, further, they are disposed in relation to the cutting edge in the manner that permits easy manipulation and, hence, the greatest saving of energy consistent with the particular function. Some handles are of a generalized nature, permitting manipulation in a variety of ways and the tool to be applied to the work from a variety of directions. In such tools the hand must be shifted frequently, and therefore the handle is of a generalized pattern that permits such shifting. The screwdriver and the chisel are examples. When the chisel is compared to the wood plane, which is nothing more than a controlled chisel, the handle is found disposed in a definite fixed manner. In the use of this tool the stroke is always the same and, hence, no shifting of the hand is required. The handle can be disposed and fashioned in such a manner that the tool can be manipulated with the least amount of energy. Another example of a precise arrangement of the grasping parts of a tool is the mowing scythe. Here the handles are disposed in a most bizarre manner, and yet they permit an ease of manipulation of the cutting edge that minimizes the fatigue of the user.

The roots of the teeth are their handles, but since the grasping mechanism is incapable of making instantaneous adjustments as is the case with the hands, the fullest efficiency and greatest power only can be developed by a maximum use of design in the relationship between teeth on the one hand and the periodontal fibers and bone on the other. But before analyzing the root form of any tooth, it is necessary to understand the mechanics by which a tooth resists forces that play upon it during function.

In teeth possessing occlusal surfaces, i.e. premolars and molars, the greatest vector of functional force is in the direction of the long axis of the tooth. This force is resisted by two major factors, both of which are contributed by the structure of the periodontium. The first one to be considered is the presence of blood and lymph vessels, which lie in great numbers between the tooth and its surrounding bony socket.

This network of fluid-containing vessels constitutes an hydraulic chamber, which helps to prevent the closely fitting tooth from being driven into its socket. Since the walls do not permit a rapid escape of the compressed fluids, considerable pressure may be built up within the socket. This best can be appreciated by the excruciating pain which accompanies the first stage of periapical abscess formation. Under normal conditions of heavy function the pressure, being momentary, is resisted without pain, but that there is a limit is attested by the gnathodynamometer. Under testing conditions, the tactile nerve endings give warning when the limit is reached.

The second and main source of resistance lies in the fibers of the periodontal ligament. For the purpose of our present discussion, it may be said that teeth are suspended in their sockets by thousands of tiny fibers which act in the manner of guy wires. These fibers do not run in direct line to the surrounding bone, but rather in curved courses. They are not elastic, but their curved courses, plus the presence between them of numerous blood and lymph vessels, permits a slight degree of motion of the tooth within the socket.

In such a tension arrangement it should be obvious that the only force that might be capable of tensing all of the fibers attached to a tooth would be one acting in the direction of the long axis. A force falling at right angles on a tooth having a root that was circular in cross-section would tense just half of the fibers. When it is recalled that the incisor teeth pass each other in function and that the cusps of the bicuspids and molars, through their inclined planes, introduce lateral forces, it becomes evident that all force is not transmitted in the line of the axis; indeed, little of it travels this course in the incisor teeth.

A post embedded in the ground, if struck from the side, will exhibit almost equal and opposite movement at the surface and at the embedded end, providing the density of the ground is the same at all depths. This means that the axis of rotation is midway of the embedded part. A tooth in its socket behaves quite differently. In the undisturbed specimen, it can be seen that the wall of the alveolus does not parallel the root surface throughout its entire extent. It is slightly wider at the crest and gradually narrows to an area about three quarters down to the root. From here to the apex it again widens slightly; thus, there is a condition of a cone sitting in an hourglass receptacle. The constricted area represents the zone of rotation. Experimental tooth movement followed by histologic study has borne this out.

When a tooth receives a force at right angles to its axis, the force is resisted almost exclusively by the fibers on the opposite side between the point of rotation and the crest of the alveolus. The greatest part of the force is taken by the fibers closest to the surface. It is therefore not surprising that the greatest concentration of fibers is found at this level. A tooth which, through periodontal disease or other cause, loses these fibers becomes very loose while a tooth which loses half of its apical end by resorption remains firm.

A tooth in function exhibits a slight degree of motion. Since the center of such motion lies a quarter of the way up the root, it follows that there must be some movement in the opposite direction at the apex. As was mentioned above, this might be indicated by the slight divergence of the walls of the socket of this area, but that the apex offers much resistance to movement is denied by the relative scarcity of the periodontal fibers attached here as well as by the profuse blood and iymph vessels supplying the tooth, which demand more room.

17.
X-Ray Studies/Cephalometry

The advantage to be gained from the utilization of roentgenograms in research on the head was pointed out by Pacini in 1922. He demonstrated to the anthropologists that accurate measurements could be made from skull x-rays more easily than from the skull itself. Pacini showed that one had only to add an object of known length to the exposed field and to employ a known object-target distance to reduce the enlarged measurement derived from the film to absolute size.

The strongest impetus toward the use of x-ray as a method of studying growth was imparted by T. Wingate Todd. An English-trained physician, with a special interest in human and comparative anatomy, he joined the medical faculty of Western Reserve University following World War I as a professor of anatomy. His clinical interests lay in the field of pediatrics, although his early investigative efforts were directed toward comparative anatomy, particularly odontology.

This culminated in the publication of his *An Introduction to the Mammalian Dentition,* the preparation of which led to the development of the Western Reserve craniostat for the precise measurement of animal skulls (Fig. 17a).

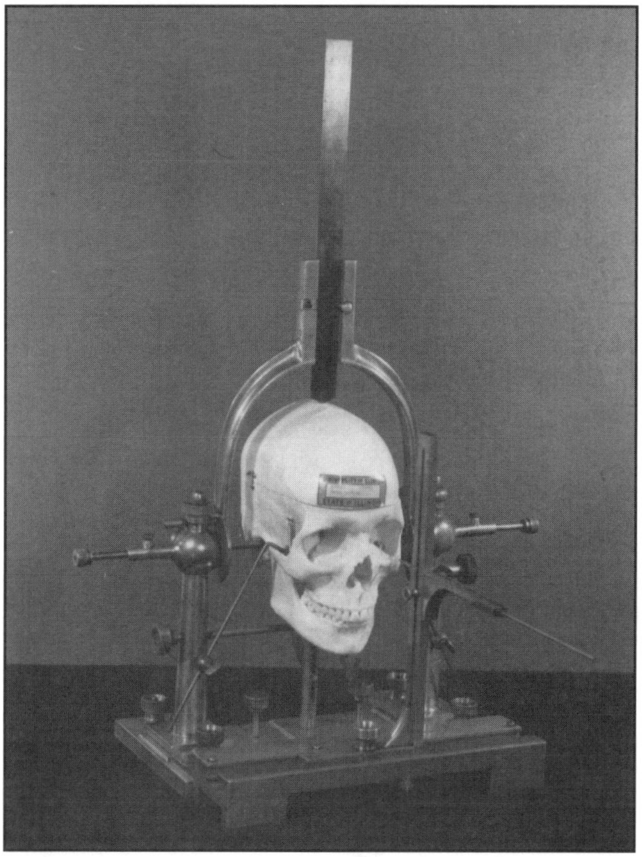

Fig. 17a. T. Wingate Todd (Western Reserve) craniostat.

Perhaps because of his intense interest in pediatric problems, Todd was one of the first to recognize the importance of growth. Medicine and dentistry, interested in the treatment of disease and abnormalities, had all but completely neglected it. Todd laid comprehensive plans to study growth by every means at his disposal. Having already gathered and prepared hundreds of skulls and skeletons from dissection rooms and morgues and having developed a standard method for x-raying the entire body, he proceeded to add these growth records to his voluminous library.

With the aid of a grant from the Brush Foundation, Todd began the study of children in Cleveland at three-month intervals beginning with the third post-natal month. After the first year the intervals were six months and from five years annually, so long as the interest of the family could be maintained. Their reward was complete medical supervision by specialists. Over the years the records of hundreds of children were collected for longitudinal study.

Early in these studies, Todd recognized that the x-ray could be put to much wider use. From the x-ray's inception, the medical clinician had employed x-rays to examine the skeleton for fractures and other morphological conditions, and for this he wanted "hard," that is, high contrast films. Todd demonstrated that it was possible to obtain vastly more information by altering the variables of exposure, e.g., time, voltage and milliamperage, and the "soft" film came into use.

It would be difficult to overemphasize the impact of Todd's laboratory on growth studies. In addition to his own contributions on incremental enlargement were those on the more subtle phenomena accompanying it, e.g., differentiation and maturation, and studies for which these were the incentive such as those of Greulich and Pyle on the hand and wrist, of Pyle and Hoerr on the knee, and of Hoerr and Frances on the ankle. Todd's earlier comparative anatomical studies culminated in Krogman's thesis *The Problem of Growth Changes in the Face and Skull as Viewed From a Comparative Study of Anthropoids and Man* in 1930.

Broadbent joined Todd's staff at Western Reserve in the early 1920s. He had received his instruction in anatomy under Todd while a dental student, and had subsequently gone to Angle to study orthodontics. There he became interested in dento-facial relations through efforts to make the facial profile visible on x-ray films by means of radiopaque substances such as bismuth paste.

Returning to Cleveland, Broadbent sought to make the derivation of measurements of the skull x-rays possible with the same accuracy as those made directly with Todd's craniostat. Succeeding in this, he turned his attention to the living head. The result was the Broadbent-Bolton roentgenographic cephalometer (Figs. 17b and 17c). Thus in 1931, a prediction made by Scammon in 1923 was fulifilled:

"The methods of roentgenography have not been applied successfully as yet to the study of postnatal skull development. All our knowledge of the subject is based either on measurements of the head in the living or on the examination of prepared skulls. The latter are often warped in drying and may be of uncertain history, consequently any description

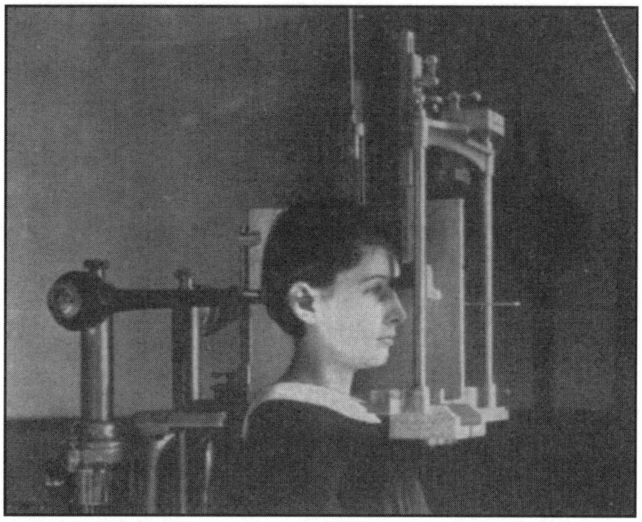

Fig. 17b. Top: Broadbent-Bolton roentgenographic cephalometer, with patient in position for taking of lateral head roentgenogram. Below: Complete Broadbent-Bolton installation showing tube assemblages and control stand.

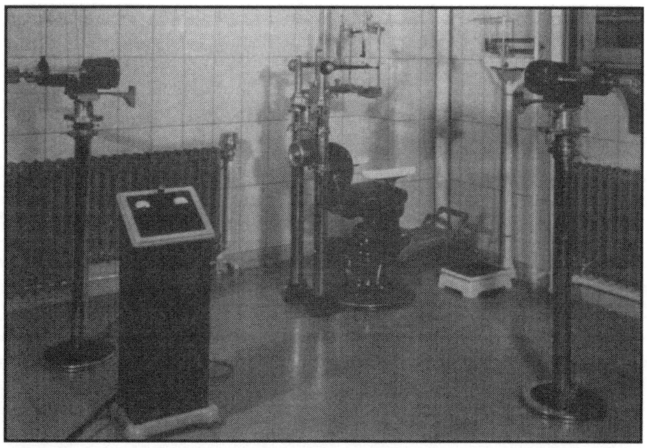

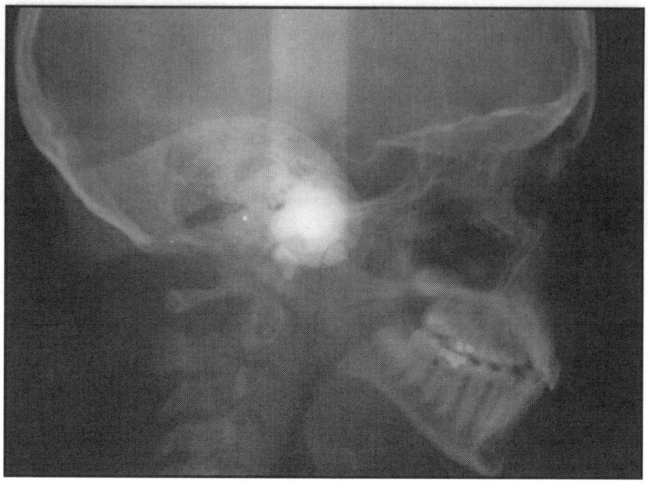

Fig. 17c. X-ray in cephalometer.

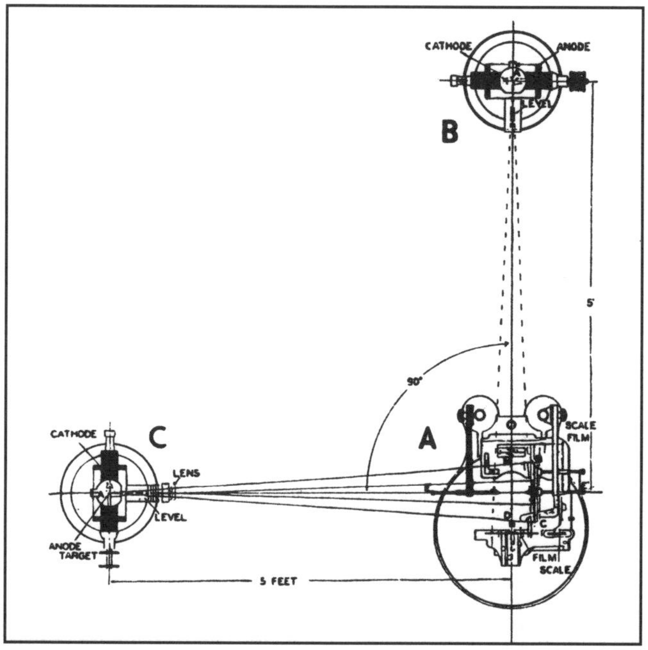

Fig. 17d. Drawing showing relation of central rays to sagittal and portion planes and to film surfaces in Broadbent-Bolton cephalometer.

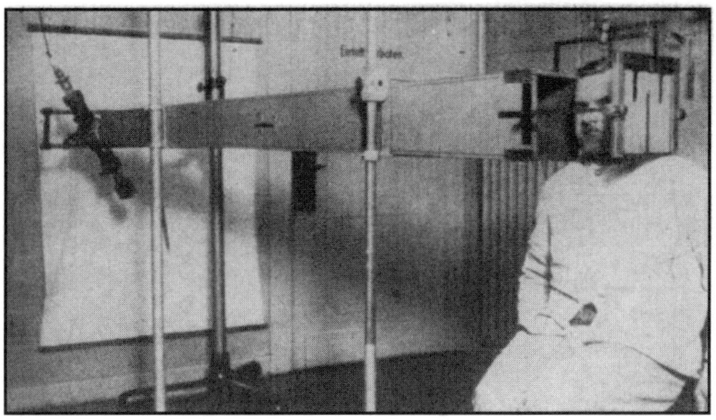

Fig. 17e. Hofrath x-ray machine.

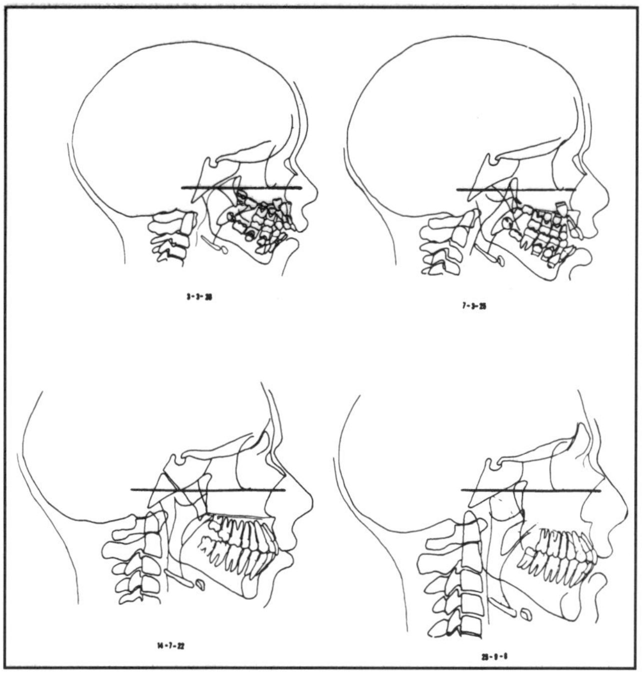

Fig. 17f. Tracings of serial cephalometric x-rays of male observed from three years, three months of age to 25 years, nine months of age.

of the process can be regarded merely as an outline subject to revision as more data are collected by modern methods." See Fig. 17d.

The same month that Broadbent published his paper "A New X-ray Technique and Its Application to Orthodontia," Hofrath of Germany published a technique to yield reproducible x-rays of the head. He employed a two-meter anode/object distance and called his method teleoroentgenography (Fig. 17e), while Broadbent employed a five-foot distance and called it cephalometric roentgenography. Hofrath was interested only in showing changes induced by surgical or prosthetic measures, and hence wanted films sufficiently undistorted to permit the superpositioning of "before and after" films. Broadbent, being interested in phenomena covering greater time intervals, desired a method that that would permit the identical placement of the head in the system regardless of age. He also wished to make it possible to take dimensions in all three planes of space, as could be done with the craniostat. To accomplish this, he employed a second tube, the anode of which was positioned five feet in back of the head-holding device. In the movable base of the head-holder, he embedded two vernier mm. scales to permit measurement of the distance of the lateral film from the midsagittal plane (M.L.) and from the frontal film to the transporionic axis (P.). The support of Broadbent's work was assumed by Mrs. Frances P. Bolton and her son, Charles B. Bolton. Through establishment of the Bolton Foundation, the collection of records followed the same schedule as that of the Brush Foundation.

When it is desired to study the changes that have taken place between different points in time, e.g., "before and after" treatment or growth stages, recourse is had to serial studies. This has become one of the most frequently employed devices of the orthodontist to show changes that have been credited to his treatment. It consists of superimposing successive tracings of films on some point, line, or angle common to all tracings. Broadbent introduced the method in 1931 and fully explained it again in 1937 in his paper, "The Face of the Normal Child." The problem he faced was the one confronting anyone desiring to measure any object: where to establish zero. See Fig. 17f.

The technique of cephalometric roentgenography as generally employed is so well-known that its review here would serve no useful purpose; but the too-literal interpretation of the evidence derived from it can be very misleading. The chief cause of such misinterpretation rests in the manner of superposing the tracings. When successive head films are superposed in the manner proposed by Broadbent, it is possible to state with assurance only that the distance between the point of superposition and some point peripheral to it has increased. The x-rays yield only overall increases and their directions; they do not reveal where the actual increases occurred. For this, one needs information from different types of investigations such as vital staining, implantation, or microscopy. Armed with qualitative information from one of these, he is in better

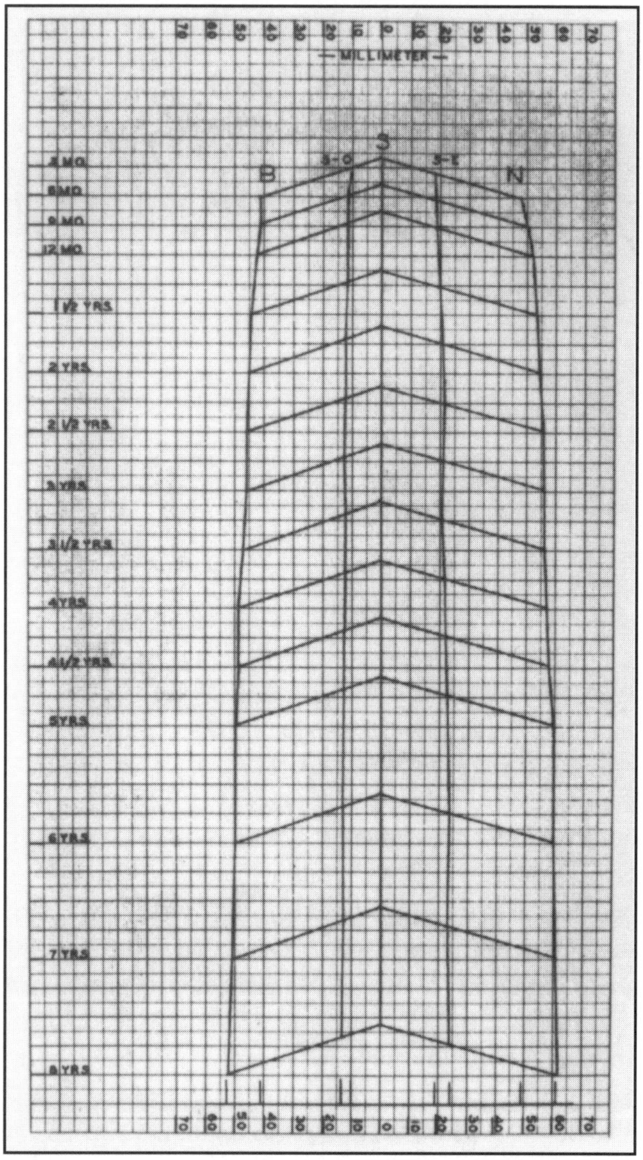

Fig. 17g. Graph representing incremental growth of cranial bone from the sixth month to the eighth year of age, mean of 21 males.

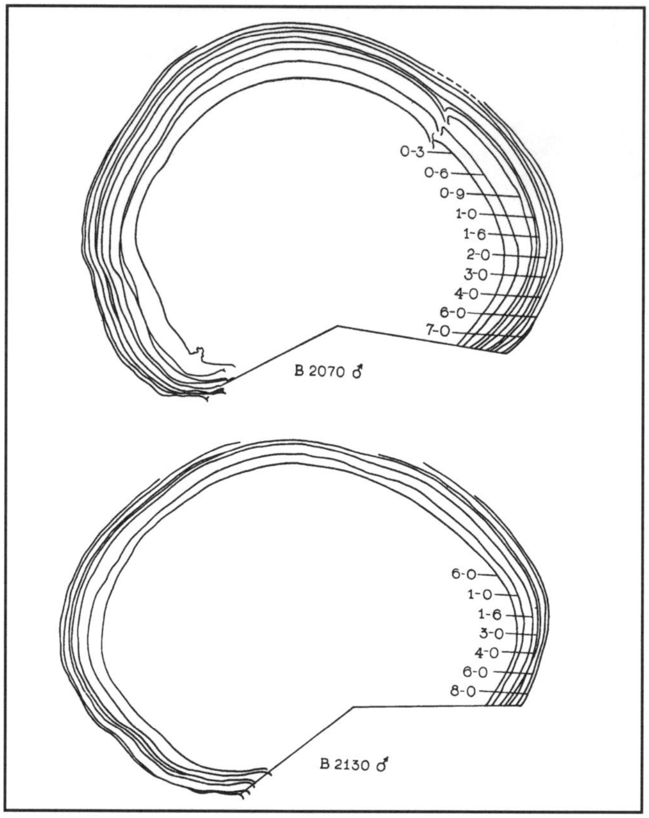

Fig. 17h. Different types of incremental growth patterns of two children, with persistence of early characteristics.

position to superpose his tracings (Figs. 17g and 17h).

When Broadbent published "A New X-ray Technique and its Application to Orthodontia" in 1931, he demonstrated the stability of sella turcica as compared with that of the ear hole, which had previously been used. His 1937 paper, "The Face of the Normal Child," showed strikingly that the point porion, representing the ear hole, travels downward and backward relative to sella turcica during growth (Fig. 17i).

The midpoint on the anterior border of foramen magnum (basion) has long been a favored point with craniologists, because it marked the point of least movement between the head and the body. However, basion could not easily be discerned on the early lateral x-ray of the head. As a posterior substitute in this same stable area Broadbent select-

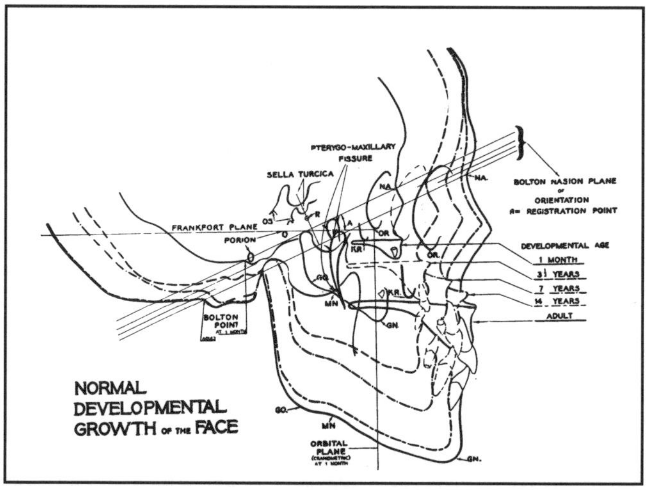

Fig 17i. Normal developmental growth of the face from Bolton study records. A=angle of Frankfort plane of the first record to the Bolton-Nasion plane of orientation. GN=gnathion. GO=gonion. KR=key ridge. NA=naison. OR=orbitale. OS=Occipito-sphenoidal suture. MN=manidbular notch.

ed a point indicating the height of the curvature of the neck of the occipital condyle where it joins the squama of the occipital bone. He called it the "Bolton point" in honor of the supporters of his work. A line connecting the right and left Bolton points crosses the middle of the foramen magnum. As the anterior terminal of the cranial base, the junction of the nasal bones with the frontal bone at the midline (nasion) was selected. A straight line drawn between nasion and the Bolton point was accepted as representing the dividing line between the brain case and face. Broadbent noted the stability of sella turcica and selected its center RSU as an additional registration point. To determine how much error might be involved in selecting the center by inspection, he asked a number of individuals to locate it on duplicate tracings, and the resulting scatter was shown to be within the area of the head of a pin. Drawing lines from the RSS point, as it is called, to both nasion and Bolton, resulted in the triangle BSN which was tentatively accepted as representing the cranial base, held to be the most stable area of the head. To adjust for growth increases in height of this triangle, a perpendicular dropped from S to the base line BN was bisected and called R, denoting registration point. Successive tracings were compared by registering on R, with the BN lines parallel. As can be seen, the orderly development of the head is clearly demonstrated qualitatively by this means.

Reading list:

Broadbent, B.H. "A new x-ray technique and its application to orthodontia." *Angle Orthodontist,* 1: 45-66, 1931.

Broadbent, B.H. "The face of the normal child," *Angle Orthodontist,* 7: 183-208, 1937.

Hofrath, H. "Bedeutung der Röntgenfern und Abstands Aufnahme für die Diagnostik der Kiefer-anomalien." *Fortschr. der Orthod.* 1: 231-258, 1931.

Pacini, A.J. "Roentgen ray anthropometry of the skull." *J. Rad.,* 230-238, 322-332, 428-426, 1922.

Todd, Thomas Wingate. *An introduction to the mammalian dentition.* St. Louis: C.V. Mosby Co., 1918.

18.
Embryological Development of the Face

Viewing the embryonic face from in front, attention is drawn to a marked depression in the center which is created by various swellings around it. At the bottom of this depression, which is the primitive stomodeum, lies the bucco-pharyngeal membrane, already rupturing to afford access to the gut.

Beneath this, and forming the lower boundary of the depression, are bilateral swellings. These represent the mandibular arches. At their most lateral and posterior parts are swellings which descend from the forebrain region and represent the maxillary processes.

At about five weeks, bilateral pits appear above the stomodeal opening. They are deepened by the swelling of their margins which form horseshoe-shaped elevations, the ends of which project downward. The medial pair are the nasomedial processes, and the lateral pair are the nasolateral processes.

The nasomedial process develops rapidly, and as the maxillary process grows medially, the two meet and eventually fuse. The nasolateral process seems to rotate upward and medially and comes in contact with the superior surface of the maxillary process to help close the naso-optic furrow and complete the housing of the eye. The two nasomedial processes fuse in the midline to form the philtrum of the upper lip, while their lateral margins continue their fusion with the maxillary processes. Failure of this last fusion results in cleft lip, which may be either unilateral or bilateral.

Thus far we have concerned ourselves with those parts which might be said to constitute the outer wall of the face. It encloses a space, the primary stomodeum, into which will grow various structures, e.g., tongue, nasal septum, and palate, the last named destined to divide it into chambers, viz., the nose and oral cavity.

From the anterior surfaces of the paired mandibular arches near the midline and in back of the stomodeum, paired swellings develop. These are the bilateral lingual swellings. By their continued growth they invade the mouth in a forward direction and ultimately fuse with each other to form the tongue. Concomitantly, from the under surface of the brain area at the midline, a process descends to form the major portion of the septum. At this stage the tongue and septum occupy most of the stomodeal space. Anteriorly, a midline projection extends backwards from the nasomedial process to complete the nasal septum above, while lower it contributes the intermaxillary element of the palate.

The palatal shelves develop from the medial surfaces of the maxillae and extend downward on either side of the tongue (Fig. 18a). As the cephalic flexure decreases, and the body straightens, the heart descends and the tongue is pulled to a lower

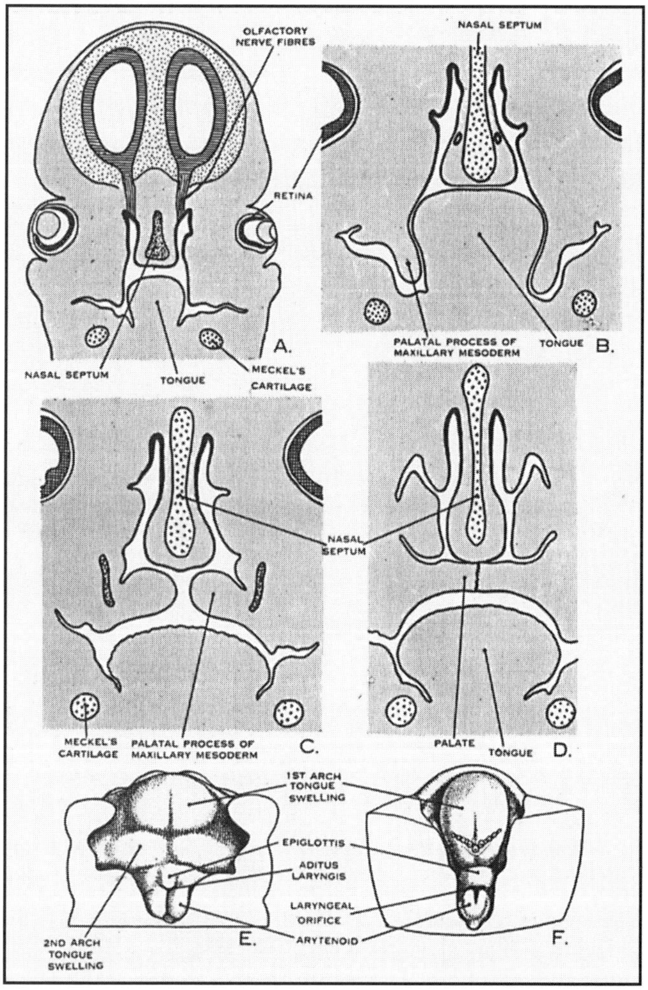

Fig. 18a. Schemes showing stages in the development of the palatal process, palate and nasal septum, A to D, and showing stages in the development of the tongue, E to F. The line of separation between the first and third arch tongue swelling is indicated by the vallate papillae.

level. This allows the palatal shelves to assume their horizontal position and they fuse with each other, forming the secondary palate. The angular interval between them anteriorly is contributed by the nasomedial process, as described above. Failure of any portions to fuse at this stage leaves an opening between the oral and nasal cavities and is known as a cleft palate.

Differentiation of Other Tissues and Organs

During the stages of development outlined above nearly all of the processes have concerned proliferation of mesenchyme, covered with epithelium. Exceptions of course are the end organs of sight and hearing, with which we are not concerned here.

One of the earliest structures to appear in the heretofore undifferentiated mesenchyme is Meckel's cartilage, which runs most of the length of the mandibular arch but does not reach the midline. It begins to resorb almost immediately from its distal end, and its proximal end becomes differentiated into the malleus and incus of the ear. Some time during this period it acts as an inducer of mandibular bone formation, as we shall see.

In the eighth embryonic week, the epithelium lining the stomodeum begins to invade the underlying mesenchyme surrounding the tongue at the level of its dorsum. This foretells the establishment of the vestibule of the mouth and dental lamina. As it proceeds outwardly it divides to send one lamina superiorly and one inferiorly. These proliferate, thereby becoming thicker, and then the central cells break down. This results in an epithelially-lined furrow, the buccal vestibule.

Before the epithelial lamina has reached the limit of its penetration of the mesenchymal wall of the stomodeum, the dental lamina has appeared. Again this seems to be a proliferation of the epithelial lamina and it follows the course of the superior surfaces of the mandibular and maxillary arches. At ten points on each of these it sends projections into the underlying mesenchyme. These are the anlagen of the deciduous teeth. They attain their cup-shaped stage by the tenth embryonic week.

Centers of ossification appear in the mandible and maxilla as early as the sixth week. That in the mandible appears to be induced by Meckel's cartilage, from one point at which it seems to start. It is possible that a similar cartilage inducer has a transitory existence in the maxilla, but it has been described only in the rat.

We see that there is a long sequence of events which must occur in a regular order before any part has completed its embryonic life or differentiation, and not until then does growth occur to any marked extent. It is a mistake to think of all embryonic processes as occurring simultaneously. Certain systems seem to have priority in growth rates over other systems, and certain parts over other parts at specific times. Thus, the central nervous system appears very early, as the neural folds, and later the neural tube differentiates on the germinal disc in front of the primitive streak. Five secondary brain vesicles develop rapidly as a further differentiation of the anterior end of the neural tube. (All are present by the fifth week.) The primitive gut does not exist until the edges of the disc are folded under and fused on the ventral side.

It is equally a mistake to think that embryological (differentiative) changes cease by the end of the third month of gestation. It is true that the body has attained its definitive form and that most of the organs and parts are present by this time. However, the teeth have still to go through their further developmental stages in fetal life and early infancy, the bones of the wrists will appear still later, and the mesenchymal tissues of the body are ready at any age to go through transformation in the interests of repair. Some types of cells, particularly of the connective tissues, retain potentialities to differentiate into highly specialized cells, for instance, into "bone builders" (osteoblasts and osteocytes). A grasp of all these facts is essential to the correct understanding of the causes and nature of abnormal growth.

Ignoring all considerations of heredity for the moment, let us assume there has been a union of two perfect cells—the male and female. As we know, the fertilized ovum is embedded in the wall of the uterus and the resulting embryo, in the higher animals at least, becomes a parasite on the mother. Nothing can reach it except through the maternal blood stream. Thus, it is very well buffered physically from the outside environment, but it should never be forgotten that the response of the mother to her environment may cause changes in the chemistry of her meabolism sufficiently to have an effect on the embryo.

These thoughts are introduced here to indicate the nature of some of the things that may lead to abnormal growth. Among damaging factors, which might become effective upon the early embryo through the blood stream of the mother and by dialysis through the placenta, may be mentioned: alcohol, narcotics, toxins from industrial poisons (lead), drugs (as in unsuccessful abortions), reductions in O_2, vitamin deficiencies, and diseases of the pregnant mother. These all might be considered as nutritional factors against which the embryo might not be sufficiently well buffered to completely overcome their handicapping influences. If this is the case, some of the vital embryological processes may be retarded or even completely inhibited. Some of these influences are only temporary (weather, disease), while others may continue throughout the entire period of gestation. How how do they act?

Any factor that is strong enough to affect the embryo in its very early stages will probably be enough to kill it and bring on miscarriage. The earlier a noxious factor becomes effective, the more severe is its influence. But if this critical stage has been passed, the effects may be shown in various defects which may range from general retardations and arrests of development to the creation of monsters. The time of occurrence of the harmful impact probably determines the degree of severity more than any other single factor. This is explainable on the following basis.

As we have seen, each part and each organ goes through certain preliminary stages, viz., initiation, proliferation, morphodifferentiation, and histodifferentiation. Then growth follows. But all parts are not at the same stage at the same time. Thus, let us imagine three parts each at a different stage when the adverse factor makes itself felt: one has completed its morphodifferentiation, one its proliferation, and one is about to be initiated. The insulting agent, working through the blood stream, acts on all of them and many bodily processes, save perhaps the purely vegetative, may become inhibited for a time. As a result, the part that has completed its morphodifferentiation and should be growing at its highest rate, loses this amount of early growth and will never make it up. It will be retarded in growth. The part which has completed its proliferation is stopped short of its morphodifferentiation and remains as a mass of embryonic cells, which may eventually break down to form cysts. The third, which is about to be initiated, never develops at all and the result is a so-called congenital absence (ear, limb, tooth).

Until comparatively recently there was little satisfactory evidence to explain the occurrence of congenital abnormalities. Many, if not all of them, were blamed on heredity. With advances in the gathering of vital statistics other factors, of environmental nature, began to assume significance, e.g., the rise in deformities following epidemics. This encouraged widespread experimental work which uncovered a wide variety of agents that might bring on deformity. But these research efforts could do no more than point to a very plausible cause and effect relationship; they did nothing to explain how they operated.

With the development of methods that made possible the analysis of the macromolecular structure of somatic cells, the geneticist was furnished with a tool that sheds new light on the matter of heriditary transmission. He was able to show that a very slight derangement in the make-up of a molecule could result in specific flaws in such matters as certain metabolic processes. These he called "inborn errors of metabolism." This line of investigation holds great promise for the elucidation of phenomena that have heretofore been almost complete mysteries.

Congenital Abnormalities of the Face

It will be recalled that the maxillary process meets and fuses with the nasomedial process of the frontal prominence to form the upper lip, and complete the outer face above the mouth opening. If there is failure of fusion here a cleft lip will result, but the defect will not necessarily involve the deeper portion of the junction. A suture can be seen in not a few newborn skulls immediately behind the incisive area indicating the boundary between the palatal shelves of the premaxilla and those of the maxillae. Failure here results in a cleft of the alveolar margin of the jaw; a cleft beyond the junction of the premaxilla and the maxilla is a cleft palate and may involve the shelves of the maxilla and palatine bones as well as the tissues of the soft palate.

It can be readily realized that all of these events do not occur simultaneously but rather in a precisely ordered sequence. This sequence had already been worked out quite thoroughly by His (in 1892) and other embryologists, but the etiology of abnormalities was laid at the door of heredity by most.

William F. Petersen at the University of Illinois devoted his research for many years to a consideration of the effects of weather (temperature, barometric pressure, and humidity) on the body's economy. He showed that even sex ratios may be influenced oy weather, many more males being conceived under certain conditions while a preponderance of females will be conceived under other conditions. For every change in the atmosphere the body must make adjustments. If the changes are sudden and extreme there always is the possibility that sufficient adjustment cannot be made. Under these circumstances disturbances of one sort or another may result. Petersen showed that under conditions of extreme weather disturbance conceptions are more apt to result in exceptional individuals and in *congenital deformities*. This also is borne out in the evolutionary principle that the greatest advances have been made during the times of greatest stress. In other words, extreme conditions result in extreme types, both superior and inferior to average.

Congenital Deformities

The heart bulge in the developing embryo completely covers the face which is forming inside the curl of the cephalic end (Fig. 18a). This makes it necessary to section or decapitate the embryo in order to see these structures, so most illustrations will show an adjoining cross-section in the general region of the thorax.

Viewed from the front, the four-week embryo presents a broad shallow depression. This is the stomodeum, the floor of which is formed by the oral plate which will rupture and provide access to the foregut. The roof of the stomodeum is formed by the vesicle of the forebrain just below the frontal prominence, which forms the most anterior aspect. On the anterior surface the placodes arebounded by horseshoe-shaped elevations which give the impression that they have sunk into the subjacent tissue and lie at the bottom of depressions: the nasal pits. The medial extensions of the horseshoes are called the nasomedial process and the lateral extensions are called the nasolateral processes. On either side of the stomodeum and caudal to the frontal prominence a large swelling grows medially and forward. This is the maxillary process, which forms the lateral parts of the upper jaw.

Caudally and ventrally to the maxillary processes a series of elevations separated by grooves appear in what will become the posterior pharyngeal wall. These paired elevations grow ventrally and medially and tend to fuse at the midline as arches enclosing the pharynx. These are the branchial arches. The most superior of these is the largest and is called the mandibular arch, because the lower jaw will be formed from it. Caudally to the mandibular arch lie the hyoid and two other arches, named merely "three" and "four." These three arches disappear later with their deeper structures giving rise to the hyoid bone and the laryngeal cartilages.

The anterior and lateral wall of the upper face is formed by a complex series of proliferations, foldings, and fusions involving the maxillary and nasal processes and their constituent tissues. The paired maxillary processes grow ventrally and medially beneath the nasolateral processes until they meet and fuse with the nasomedial processes. Failure of fusion at this junction results in cleft lip and/or palate. Further medial growth of the maxillary process carries them toward the midline until they seem to squeeze the bilateral nasomedial processes into a single midline structure. Their upward extension lateral to the nasolateral process permits fusion with the frontal prominence and completes the enclosure of the eye. This largely completes the tissues of the face from which the nose, cheeks, and lips will arise.

The nasal pits become progressively deeper by the growth of the nasal processes around them until they eventually rupture to afford communication between the outside and the upper part of the stomodeum.

If attention were directed to the inner aspect of the structures just described, it would be found that the two nasomedial processes fuse to become a single intermaxillary element which will house the incisor teeth. Both this structure and the maxillary process give origin to inwardly directed palatal shelves at a level below that of the internal nasal openings. Those of the maxilla are directed directly obliquely downward on either side of the tongue, making it appear that that organ would prevent their joining, as it is sometimes said to do. Normally the tongue is withdrawn from between these processes as the cephalic flexure decreases and the straightening of the body draws the visceral structures downward. The palatal shelves are thus able to rotate upward into correct approximation to close the palatal vault.

There is not complete agreement on where the centers of ossification first appear in the maxillae, but it seems certain that there are separate centers in the maxillary and intermaxillary processes. These centers enlarge until they join with adjacent centers. The resulting junctions may be obliterated or remain for a longer or shorter period as sutures. The most evident of these lies in the midsagittal plane where it separates the premaxillae, the maxillae, and the shelves of the palatine bones. Complete closure of this suture does not usally occur before the end of puberty and may be delayed well into adult life. A patent mid-palatal suture makes possible the orthodontic procedure of palate splitting that has been reintroduced in recent years.

Reading list:

Hamilton, W.J., Boyd, J.D, Mossman, H.W. *Human Embryology.* Baltimore: The Williams & Wilkins Co., a William Wood Book, 1945.

19.
Embryological Development of the Dental Apparatus

Before proceeding with a consideration of the phylogeny of the dental apparatus, it will be helpful to review certain aspects of embryology, because ontogeny recapitulates phylogeny to a remarkable degree and the stages of embryologic development have been studied for a considerable period of time. The present discussion will be limited to the formation and disposition of the three germ layers of the main body cavities.

Following its implantation in the wall of the uterus, the fertilized ovum undergoes rapid cell division to form a mass of cells called the morula. Fluid gathers inside the peripheral cells of this mass and separates them from the rest, except at one place. The resulting cavity is called the blastocele, and the attached clump of cells is called the inner cell mass. The cells of the periphery in contact with the cells of the uterine lining are called the trophoblast.

Next, a second accumulation of liquid takes place in the inner cell mass resulting in the formation of another vesicle within it, the amniotic cavity. Thus, two cavities come to lie opposite each other separated only by several cell layers. The cells of this partition which face the amniotic cavity are ectodermal, those facing the yolk sac (formerly blastocele) are endodermal, and the cells which lie between the two layers become primitive mesoderm. The cellular partition is the embryonic disc, destined to become the embryo.

It is helpful if one now imagines the result of a continuing accumulation of fluid in the amniotic sac. Being confined within the trophoblast, its expansion expresses itself outward in all directions from the edge of the embryonic disc so that it not only comes to form an almost complete lining for the trophoblast, but also tends to curl the periphery of the disc down.

The disc might be said to lie on the surface of the yolk sac at this stage, and important changes are taking place on its upper (amniotic) surface. Rapid proliferation occurs at the edge of the sac and a streak appears which establishes the axis of the disc. The epithelium on the immediate sides of the streak proliferates until a v-shaped neural groove results. About this time the ectoderm and endoderm, which compose the partition between the amniotic and the yolk sacs, are separated by embryonic mesoderm. Proliferation of this tissue between the neural groove in the back and the yolk sac in front results in a cylindrical rod of cells, the notochord. This is the primitive vertebral column.

The edges of the neural groove curl toward each other, merge, and form a tube of epithelial cells which is cut off from the surface epithelium by the invasion of mesoderm. A similar invasion isolates the notochord and forms the neural groove and yolk sac.

At the anterior or cephalic end of the neural groove, three dilations appear in its walls. In order from behind to forward these are the anlagen or precursors of the hind brain, the mid brain, and the forebrain. Their edges, like those of the groove, curl toward each other to fuse and form the three primary brain vesicles.

Up to this point it has been advantageous to describe events as though the primitive disc were a flat structure. Now it must be recalled that it lies on the surface of the yolk sac, which diminishes in size as the amnionic sac continues to increase. The disc between them, growing at a lower rate, becomes curved both cephalocaudally and bilaterally as it conforms to the shrinking yolk sac. The lateral edges of the disc curl medially, meet, and fuse at the ventral midline, ectoderm to ectoderm, endoderm to endoderm, and in the middle region mesoderm to mesoderm. At the cephalic and caudal ends the mesoderm is lacking, so here ectoderm and endoderm also meet.

The embryo can now be thought of as a tube, with the meeting of the two edges resulting in the establishment of the primitive gut. By this time the swelling amnion has completely enveloped the embryo everywhere except in one area of the ventral midline toward the caudal end. Here the yolk sac has been compressed into a tube which is embedded in mesenchymal tissue. It communicates with the gut and forms part of the body stalk and, eventually, the umbilical cord.

The portion of the disc lying between the vesicles of the forebrain is one of the places at which the mesodermal layer is missing and endoderm and ectoderm meet. This is the buccopharyngeal membrane. By this time, the swelling of the amnion has resulted in a ventral bending of the embryo at its ends to form the cephalic and caudal folds or flexures. This brings the head parts down to an almost right angle relation to the axis of the primitive gut so that the endothelium of the buccopharyngeal membrane is brought into approximation with that of the foregut. The second mesoderm-deficient area (cloacal membrane) lies at the other end of the embryo and results from the apposition of the endoderm of the disc and that of the hind gut. The rupture of these two membranes establishes communication between the two ends of the gut and the outside. The embryology of the face and dental apparatus will be considered under their appropriate sections.

This chapter, beyond serving as a review of essential material that is often neglected in dental education, also is intended to emphasize the relatively few basically simple embryologic phenomena that result in such a wide variety of organs and parts. Beginning as a flat disc, the embryo is transformed into a complex three-dimensional body by relatively few processes which are repeated over and over again with only slight variations to produce strikingly different structures and relations.

The three original germ layers are of primary interest, each with its own specific potential for development of its future functions. The ectoderm is primarily protective, forming the outer covering of the body and the lining of those apertures (mouth and anus) formed by infoldings of the outer surface. The endoderm lines internal cavities and channels, and the mesoderm lying between the other two contributes to their support.

The first observable class of processes is cellular proliferation. This appears at first to be a random increase of cells in all directions resulting in spherical forms such as the morula, but it is soon modified in such a way as to form a layer. Further alterations are brought about by localized differences in cellular proliferation of all of the germ layers to produce such structures as the neural crest, the thickening of the endoderm to form the notochord, and that of the mesoderm to form the primitive segments.

The most conspicuous embryologic processes are the foldings of the layers which insure the correct approximation of tissues in spite of their extreme differences in morphology and relations. The simplest of these is the curling together of edges of a single layer to form a structure such as the neural canal. When the three germ layers are involved as in the enclosing of the primitive gut the process is similar, except that three layers must meet precisely and each fuse with its corresponding layer of the opposite side.

Considerably more complicated are the processes in the head where provision must be made for the establishment of communication between the body and the environment as required for the mouth, the nose, the eyes, and the ears. It will be recalled that there was an area in the embryonic disc forward of the anterior brain vesicle where mesoderm does not develop and ectoderm and endoderm meet. This is the buccopharyngeal membrane, or oral plate.

As the amniotic sac continues to swell, the cephalic end of the embryo is progressively flexed until this plate is finally carried down and around onto the ventral surface. This brings it into approximation with the end of the foregut and, there being no mesoderm present between them, the plate perforates and the endoderm of the membrane and that of the gut join.

In a somewhat analogous manner communication is established for the nose, eyes, and ears, each by the approximation of a highly specialized end organ area of the ectoderm and the internal embryonic tissues in the absence of intervening mesoderm. Perforation follows wherever ectoderm and endoderm are approximated.

Unlike the structures considered thus far the heart develops ventrally and when it has attained its early tubular form, it lies immediately below the foregut. As it grows it produces a significant ventral bulge that faces the ventral surface of the forebrain vesicle as a result of the cephalic flexure. By this time the embryo has attained almost a semicircular form when viewed from the lateral aspect, but it soon begins to straighten as the flexions decrease.

In the team approach to the management of congenital anomalies of the facial region, the prominent role of the orthodontist makes it imperative that he be well informed of its embryological development.

20. The Growth of Abnormal Head Patterns

Principles of Development

Early embryonic processes are strikingly similar whether we think in terms of entire animal bodies or of individual organs and parts. Indeed, they are so alike that only an expert could detect the differences between a lizard, a bird, a horse, and a human, in the early stages. Specific human features of the head and face, for instance, are not recognizable before the seventh or eighth week. Much the same holds true of the early development of organs, for while there are specific differences in the early primordia, there are certain characteristic stages through which they all seem to go. And in the early developmental stages of each organ we find a recapulation of the early development of the body, just as the body of each new individual recapitulates the phylogenetic development or evolution of the face.

Initiation

Obviously, every new process, whether of the whole or one of its parts, must have a beginning. It must be initiated. Thus, in the case of the new being we have the fertilization of the ovum, or the joining of two cells, which individually have no significance. United they carry the thread of life and of evolution. Except under the microscope, this process of initiation can only be detected after it has started on the second stage.

Proliferation

Immediately following the initiation of a formative process there is a rapid increase in the number of cells through an intense mitotic activity. In the case of the embryo this leads to the development of the morula or mulberry mass, while in tooth formation it leads to the bud stage. Although the cells have increased greatly in numbers, they are seemingly identical in structure and form.

Histodifferentiation

This stage shows the beginning of the development of differences between the involved various groupings taking place. In the case of the morula, we find the cells gathering themselves together at one area on the inside of its limiting membrane while fluid occupies the remaining space. Then the cells arrange themselves in a layer and we say the ectoderm has come into being—a disc of cuboidal cells. Almost immediately thereafter comes the formation of another layer beneath the first—the endoderm—and finally, a third appears between them—the mesoderm. The three primary germ layers have appeared. In the case of the tooth the "morula" is the bulb-like mass of cells which descends from the dental lamina and, like the morula, it is composed of a mass of cells, all of which are alike. Soon afterward, the deepest cells of this mass become differentiated into cuboidal forms and arrange themselves in a layer at the bottom of the sac, which in the meantime has buckled inward. At this buckled area there occurs a differentiation of the cells lying in contact with it, but on the outside, i.e., on the concave side of the cup. These cells, mesodermal in origin, also become cuboidal and arrange themselves as a layer in contact with the first. The bell stage has been reached.

Morphodifferentiation

Not until this stage is reached do we have any idea of what is forming, and even here it must be well advanced before we can be certain because of the great similarities that exist between dissimilar organs. The embryo, in the stage of histodifferentiation, has become a disc lying on the surface of a nutritive sac. It now begins to show certain changes which will give it three-dimensional characteristics.

This is not the place for a detailed description of general embryological processes, but certain things should be pointed out. The embryonic disc enlarges rapidly, more in length than in width, and a dimple-like structure appears in the middle of it (the primitive node and pit). As though flowing from this point a groove or trough appears, which is the forerunner of the central nervous system. At the most anterior part of this trough the brain vesicles will be formed.

There are two areas where mesoderm does not separate the ectoderm and endoderm. One of these lies just forward of the brain area and the other just in back of the neural groove.

In the meantime, the lateral edges of the disc have curled downward as though to enclose a part of the underlying yolk-sac. As these edges fuse at the ventral midline they form a tube, the primitive gut. By a flexing of the head and tail ends of the disc the two-layered areas are carried into such positions that they close the two ends of the tube. They will eventually perforate, establishing communication between the gut and the outside.

Following the complete closure of the gut, a swelling appears in the ventral wall. It is the cardiac eminence, which denotes the site of heart and liver development. The forebrain is almost in contact with this swelling and on this approximating surface the anlagen of the facial structures appear. To view them it is necessary to remove the head.

21. Preface to Growth

The student's comprehension of the phenomena of growth can be broadened by an acquaintance with the methods used to study it. The methods have been diverse: observational, experimental, physical, chemical, gross and microscopic, qualitative, and quantitative, each beginning at a simple level and becoming more sophisticated as it was refined by subsequent investigators. Occasionally, a concept based on findings derived from one method has not agreed with the findings from another method.

The erratic progress of knowledge in the field of growth makes it difficult to decide whether to consider it as a whole on a chronologic basis or on the basis of the evolution of the methods used in its study. The latter has been used in this book.

Paleontology and Anthropology

The publication of Darwin's *The Origin of Species* in 1859 marked the beginning of a revolution in biological thinking. It also offered justification for acknowledgement of paleontology as a scientific discipline. Without going into the field it should be pointed out that certain concepts originating from it have influenced subsequent biological research. The chief concept was that present animal forms are descendants of earlier forms which had undergone random changes resulting in the present status. Much of the contributing evidence consisted of bones and teeth excavated by paleontologists. W.K. Gregory has been outstanding for his elucidation of the paleomorphology of the skull and his knowledge about the muscles of mastication, and his best known text is *Our Face from Fish to Man* (Fig. 21a).

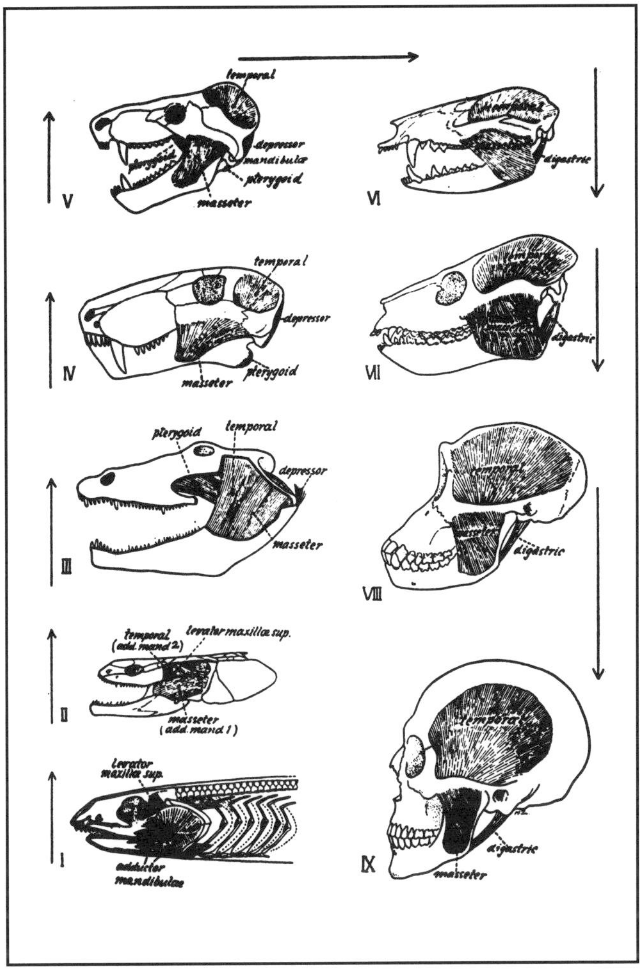

Fig. 21a. Relocation of muscles of mastication in the course of evolution.

Gregory credits Williston for the formulation of the law which bears his name. Williston states, "it is also a law of evolution that the parts of an organism tend toward reduction in number with the fewer parts greatly specialized in function just as the most perfect machine is that which has the fewest parts and each part most highly adapted to the special function it has to subserve." He pointed out that the most primitive reptile had no fewer than 72 separate bones in the skull while the human skull had only 22 bones exclusive of the inner ear bones. It is thought this reduction in number has been caused in part by the actual loss of certain bones, in part by the fusion of contiguous bones and in part by the remaining bones becoming more adapted for special use.

The skeleton of the body has only to increase proportionately in size and strength as it progresses from a prenatal to an adult pattern. Consisting of a collection of almost independent parts, the body is not subject to as many special, vital, and functional demands as the cranial skeleton. This part has witnessed the gathering together of the brain, the end organs of the the special senses (except the tactile), and the portals for entry of food and oxygen. Adding further to the complexity of analysis and the interaction among tissues, the skeletal system is made up almost entirely of mesenchymal derivatives, while ectoderm, endoderm, and mesoderm play significant roles in the head.

Each of the special sense organs seems to have developed independently from a different area in the brain, and all were supported by their own mesenchymal tissue. Gregory called them "branchial baskets." Eventually they were gathered in a protective sheath with contributions from various units, including the brain. The earliest skulls consisted of groups of bony plates. Numerous and simple in form, they were destined to be reduced to the present number, becoming more complicated in form and structure by adaptation. All were membranous bone.

But these surface structures were not the only precursors to the mammalian cranial skeleton. Other structures lying internally to the surface had functions to support the brain and special sense organs and to provide stress pathways against the forces of environment and movement. These internal bones differed from the dermal bones in derivation, being preformed in cartilage from the most anterior portion of the vertebral system. They clustered around the vertebral canal and in the mammalian skull by the basilar part and foramen magnum of the occipital bone, the body and parts of the greater and all of the lesser wings of the sphenoid bone, and the cribriform plate of the ethmoid bone. Situated posterolaterally are the cartilaginous auditory capsules.

The membranous bones may be looked upon as a protective shield enclosing the brain and the end organs of the special senses, a function they indeed do serve. In addition, most of these bones have become adapted to contribute to more than a single function by modification of their structure or by combining with adjacent structures. A few examples will illustrate this. As late as birth the temporal bone is shown to be separated into its component parts, viz. squama, petrous, mastoid, and tympanic. The sphenoid and presphenoid are still apart as also are the two halves of the frontal bone. These represent fusion of adjacent bones.

The maxilla and mandible represent bones that have acquired dominance over others in their group and have displaced them. The maxilla contributes most of the lower half of the lateral wall and the floor of the nasal cavity.

Due to its rigid nature and ready accessibility to post-mortem study, the skeletal system has claimed most of the attention for the student and investigator of growth. An early case in point was the study by Keith and Campion (1922) entitled "A Contribution to the Mechanism of Growth of the Human Face." Their study consisted of superpositioning of outlines of skulls, areas of skulls, and individual bones, and they were led to the conclusion that growth of the tissue between bones forced them apart. As has been noted previously, Brash believed "the units of growth are the bones themselves and not the sutures that connect them." These were conclusions on quantitative data, and vice-versa. Here one method revealed "how much" but not "where," and the other showed "where" but not "how much."

The Skeleton

The skeleton has come to be considered the chief determinant of the form and size of the body, as well as the form and location of its functional parts, in much the same way the framework of a house determines locations of doors, windows, and the plumbing and heating system. But, as will be seen, the opposite is true in the living body: primacy does not reside in the supporting system.

The body should be regarded as a collection of systems whose common function is to maintain life. All vital functions are controlled by soft tissue which requires specific conditions of size, location, and potential for growth and modification in the interests of procurement and conservation of energy. The skeleton thus represents a response to the demands of the soft tissue for support wherever that has been advantageous. This has been present in one form or another in all living things from the unicellular organism onward. The support was originally an intracellular component, but as increasing demands were placed on the cells from environmental forces extracellular components such as collagen fiber, cartilage, and bone were developed. The newly formed component did not lose connection with their origin, the intra- and extracellular elements being continuous.

The supporting framework of the body consists of collagen mainly in the form of densely packed fibers. Specific areas of the framework are infiltrated by inorganic salts to become bones. Each of these areas has a special form for its species, and each has received a name and become treated as a distinct unit. Together the units constitute the skeleton.

How could such a complicated mosaic of calcified units, all enlarging at the same time, each according to its own pattern, maintain proportionality while it grew? This does raise questions on the legitimacy of conclusions based on the study of individual bones. Perhaps it is justified as follows: If the two femurs are examined after one has been incinerated to ash and the other demineralized, they are identical in size and form. One represents the living and the other then the non-living component of the skeleton. The living part is composed of both intra and extracellular components, each unit being connected by sutures or synchondroses. It is then feasible to think of the skeleton as a continuum of collagen, and it is in this continuum that the pattern of development seems to reside. A young fetus gives little indication of bone, yet its conformation is the same as though it were supported by a skeleton.

The soft tissues of the body grow interstitially by cell proliferation and the elaboration of intercellular substance. Bone on the other hand can grow or change only by additions or subtractions from surfaces. Yet bone is one of the most responsive tissues to environmental forces, as has been stated by Wolf in his law:

"Any change in the form or function of a bone or of its function alone is followed by changes in its internal architecture and secondary alterations in its external form according to mathematical laws."

The responses to which Wolf referred are not those one would expect from inanimate structures which would be distorted internally as well as externally and reflect the reflection of the distorting force. Force applied to a living bone causes a response by rearrangement of all of its structural elements in such a way as to make it resistant to the distorting force. In short, bone responds against force. This has been a property of bone since earlier forms as shown by the skeleton in a sponge being arranged to best resist the action of waves in the usual direction from which they come. If the sponge is detached from its anchorage and reattached in a different direction, its spicules become reoriented to the new waves.

Reading list:

Darwin, Charles. *The Origin of Species.* New York. Grammercy, 1998.

Keith, A., and Campion, G.C. "A Contribution to the Mechanism of Growth of the Human Face," *International Journal of Ortho., Oral Surgery, and Radiology*, 8: 607-633, 1922.

22. Bone Growth

Early Studies on Bone Growth

The first work that could rightfully be called scientific on the matter of bone growth dates back to 1736. The circumstances are described by Sir Arthur Keith in the following passage.

"Some time in the summer of 1736 a calico printer of the City of London entertained to supper John Belchier, a promising young and inquiring surgeon, and all unwittingly introduced him at the same time to a method of unravelling some of Nature's great secrets. The method to which Belchier was thus introduced was that of vital staining, one by which certain elements of the body can be picked out by distinctive colors while they are still living. The calico printer was an economical man and used the madder soaked bran from his dye vats to feed pigs. The pigs he used to feed to his friends. It was a joint of this madder fed pork that was placed before the young surgeon then in his thirtieth year and just elected to the staff of Guy's Hospital. It was but natural that a young man already a Fellow of the Royal Society and a contributor to its philosophical transactions should have his curiosity aroused by the ruddy color of the bones of the madder fed pork and that he should resolve on returning to his home to make further inquiries before bringing this strange matter to the notice of the Fellows of the Society. He desired, first of all, to make certain that it was madder and no other substance which stained living bones and hence he began to feed some of his fowls with madder. One cock subjected to this treatment by force, for fowls refuse food mixed with madder, died at the end of a sixteen days' course; the bones were stained, even those of the densest structure. Early in the autumn he made a communication to the Royal Society which was subsequently printed in its transactions."

Belchier never carried his investigations any further, being fully satisfied with having called the attention of the society to the peculiar property of bone to pick up this organic dye. Three years later, however, another man, Duhamel, a French squire trained as an attorney but with an insatiable curiosity about Nature, had Belchier's paper called to his attention. Duhamel was a member of the French Academy of Science. He repeated the work Belchier had done on fowls, and having satisfied himself that this was a phenomenon that could be experimentally produced, he made a communication to the French Academy under the title, "On a root which stains bones red." However, Duhamel had the imagination to see that he had in his hands a potent tool for unravelling some of the mysteries of bone growth and metabolism. He accordingly set to work and over the next two decades experimentally explained a great many of these phenomena so fully that little has been added since that time.

One of his first findings, published in 1741, was that only certain parts of bones are stained by madder, and further, that young bones stain more deeply than old bones. He fractured the bones of fowl and noticed that the repair area, that is, the callus, was peculiarly susceptible to reception of the dye. Hence, the bone was not necessarily correlated with the age of the animal; any new bone would pick up the dye. His next experiment, and one which undoubtedly resulted from his observations of fractures, led to his alternate feeding and withholding of the dye in growing animals. After a period of non-feeding the bones were clear or unstained and this made it appear that the dye might have been dissipated or absorbed. However, upon sectioning such bones he obtained a picture of one layer of bone on another, the unstained layers masking the stained layers that lay beneath them. From this he postulated the idea that a bone grows like a tree and the periosteum is the cambion layer.

He next turned his attention to the growth of bones in length. He was aware of the fact that benchmarks in trees remained at exactly the same distance from each other. In other words, there was no extension or increase in distance between them. Applying the same techniques to the study of long bones he drilled holes in the shafts of them and kept the holes in the bones open by inserting silver eyelets. Upon sacrifice of the animal he discovered that there was no increase in the distance between these inserts, and he therefore stated that bones grew only at their ends; there was no increase of bone within the body or diaphysis. He did not mention the role played by the epiphyseal lines and did not postulate on the exact place where additions in length occurred.

One other experiment of Duhamel deserves to be mentioned here. He had noticed that if a wire was tied around the trunk of a growing tree it became embedded gradually within the substance of the trunk. Applying this same technique to a growing bone, he found that the wire came to be embedded in a similar way in the substance of the shaft, or if permitted to go long enough, might be found in the medullary cavity. He stated on the basis of these findings that there was expansion in the bone material which ultimately led to the wire being found in the center of the bone. In this he was, of course, in error and it was John Hunter who gave us our knowledge as to how the phenomenon discovered by Duhamel could actually be explained.

Until recently, concepts of how bone grows or changes rested largely on evidence derived from vital staining and occular microscopy. Both of these methods have seemed to restrict bone activity to surface depositions and resorptions of surfaces. Originally the activity was conceived to be an additive phenomenon on only the outer surface. This was the opinion of Duhamel, foremost of the early experimenters with madder. Although convinced that a long bone grew in thickness by the laying down of successive layers of bone on its outer surface, he also believed that its medullary cavity increased in size by an expansion of the shaft, i.e., some sort of interstitial growth. By inserting eyelets in the shafts of long bones and noting that they did not move apart as the bone grew, he demonstrated that bone increased in length only by growth at its ends. He missed the significance of the epiphyses. It remained for John Hunter to demonstrate that deposition was accompanied by resorption, thus explaining the increase in size of the medullary cavity. In this manner a bone was always kept trimmed to its "just proportions," as he said.

Almost 30 years after Duhamel's first work, another man destined to make great contributions to the knowledge of bone physiology, John Hunter, published his classic *Treatise on the Natural History of Human Teeth* (1771). Hunter was fully aware of Duhamel's work and accepted most of it. He did a great deal of his work, however, on pigs — a larger animal and one which of course presented jaws and teeth for study. One of the first matters which intrigued him was the behavior of the shafts of long bones, which had been studied by Duhamel as noted above. Previously, he had been intrigued by a phenomenon that undoubtedly had been noticed for countless generations pertaining to the loss of the deciduous teeth and to the eruption of their permanent successors. Strange as it may seem, it was Hunter who first pointed out the fact that when a deciduous tooth was lost, there was a complete absorption of its roots as well as of the alveolar bone that held it. This observation is thought to have focused his attention on the matter of bone absorption, and his study of the shattered bones which he had opportunity to study as a war surgeon led him to view the living body not only as a builder but also as a scavenger of those parts that were no longer needed. With this type of background, it was Hunter who postulated the idea that as a bone grew it was constantly being remodelled, and that the process of bone absorption was just as important to the economy of skeleton building as was that of deposition.

We are indebted to Hunter for the first accurate description of the growth processes of the mandible which make it possible for the dental arch to receive and accommodate three permanent molars in back of the deciduous arch. His madderized pig specimens revealed clearly that growth of the lower jaw in the pig was characterized by heavy depositions of bone at the posterior margin of the ascending ramus and by corresponding absorptions on the anterior margin of the coronoid process. In addition to these sites of change, there also was lively deposition of bone on the crest of the alveolar process. He pointed out the fact that each of the molars as it ascends in eruption takes up a position in relation to the anterior margin of the coronoid process identical to that of the tooth anterior to it at the time of *its* eruption. That is, the second deciduous first, second, and third permanent molars all bear the same relation to the ramus at the time of their eruption. On the basis of these findings Hunter announced that after the eruption of all of the deciduous teeth the dental arch of the human "Never became the arc of a larger circle but only more projecting forward."

The increase in the width of the mandible and maxilla he demonstrated to be a matter of surface deposition on the outside with a corresponding absorption on the inside, and he strongly insisted that bone growth was entirely a matter of surface apposition and resorption, and in this manner bones were kept trimmed to an economical balance regardless of the age stage at which one studied them.

It should not be inferred from what has been said here that Hunter was a blind follower of Duhamel. He had used Duhamel's method and had verified his findings, but when it came to the matter of the interpretation of the agent responsible for bone desposition he tended to follow Haller. Haller was the advocate of the idea that it was the blood system that led to bone growth. Duhamel, as has been noted, was of the opinion that the periosteum was the active and indispensible agent. It was at this early date that this controversy began, and it has continued down to the present day. Both schools, however, are insistent on the fact that growth is not interstitial—it is purely a surface phenomenon.

In 1864, Humphries of England checked Hunter's findings on the mandible by another method. He drilled a hole midway through the ascending ramus and encircled the anterior and posterior halves with silver wires. He then permitted the animals to complete their growth before sacrificing them. Upon subsequent examination it was found that the posterior wire was completely embedded in the body of the ramus, whereas the anterior wire had been sloughed off in the soft tissues anterior to the coronoid process.

In 1924 Brash repeated Hunter's work on the pig, feeding these animals with madder. In addition to completely verifying Hunter's finding on the sites of growth, namely posterior border of the ramus and alveolar process, he carried his investigations into the upper face and attempted to elucidate the manner in which the more complex upper face grew. Among other matters which he studied was that of tooth eruption and migration.

It requires but a moment's reflection to realize that if the mandible were increasing in width by a deposition on its outer surface and a resorption on its inner surface, that the lingual roots of the teeth eventually would be exposed next to the tongue. By making sections through the jaws in those areas, Brash demonstrated that the alveolus should be considered as an external surface of the mandible and maxilla. Thus, in addition to those areas of deposition on the outside of the bone proper, he found that there was active deposition of bone within the alveolus on all surfaces which faced the outside and corresponding areas of absorption on those surfaces which faced lingually. In this manner the teeth were kept in the same relative relations to the bone which held them. The gradual increase in height of the mandible through growth at its alveolar process was accompanied in a similar way by depositions of bone in the floor of the alveolus, which permitted the teeth to follow the upward growth of the bone.

We must now retrace our steps somewhat to the decade which followed 1838 when men first came to realize that the body was made up of units of atoms to which the name "cells" has come to be applied. In the field of bone growth from the cellular standpoint, the man who probably did more to elucidate some on the cellular processes was Goodsir. Goodsir had from his youth onward studied some of the lower marine forms of life, the lowly hydra for example, and by the time he was ready to begin work on bone he was an expert in the use of the new research instrument, the compound achromatic microscope, that had been perfected by Lord Lister's father. By the time he was ready to study bone, Goodsir had already studied the building of the skeleton of sponges and had noted the tiny animal-like creatures that were responsible for this phenomenon. Goodsir made some of the earliest observations on the epiphyseal lines of long bones, and here he found a striking similarity between the cartilage cells as they grouped themselves into ranks and gradually became bone-forming spicules, to the activities that he had previously observed in the formation of sponge skeletons. He traced the transformation of the primary cartilage spaces until they became Haversian canals lined by cells which he regarded as the descendants of the cartilage previously noted. He saw further how the corpuscles of the Haversian canals became included within the bone and apparently remained alive as the living constituents of the bone. Thus, he disproved Hunter's ideas that it was blood which caused bone growth and lymphatics which caused its destruction, and showed that both of these activities were the responsibility of the cell.

On sectioning the jaws of animals fed on madder, Brash showed that the walls of the alveolar sockets should be regarded as external bony surfaces subject to the same additive and subtractive changes. These changes accompanied shifts in the spatial positions of the root of the tooth leading to the maintenance of the proportional relationship between tooth and jaw. These findings, and those derived from the study of bony canals for blood vessels, gubernacular cords, marrow spaces, and sinuses, have demonstrated the presence of osteoblasts and osteoclasts on bony surfaces undergoing deposition and resorption. Deposition seems to take place on all internal and external surfaces facing the direction a bone is growing, with resorptions on surfaces facing the opposite direction. Thus, if such structures are thought of as inclusions within a bone, they give the impression that they are drifting through the bone in the same direction as its growth, at rates slightly different from those on the outer surfaces.

In addition to the changes which contribute to the increase in size of a bone, there are more subtle alterations in its structured elements known as remodeling. These include the process of area relocation, reshaping, resizing, and also the results of surface phenomena. Unfortunately, the word "surface" is generally taken to mean the external surface, and this has led to oversimplification of the concept of bone growth and remodeling. Perhaps an analogy would be helpful here:

If the reader will picture a profile x-ray of a young mandible and imagine its trabecular structure drawn on a sheet of rubber, one can easily realize how its pattern would be increased in size by stretching at the right points. Not only would its total size be increased, but also each trabecular space would be altered proportionately. The result of growth would be the same proportional increase in all parts, except that the change would have increased by localized deposition and resorption instead of merely stretching a rubber sheet. Viewed independently, each trabecular space must be conceived as presenting internal surfaces, and it is these surfaces that are subject to depositions and resorptions.

Changes in bone require the presence of cells—osteoblasts for deposition and osteoblasts for resorption. Some of the former become embedded in their own deposits of bone and remain as bone cells (osteocytes) still in communication with adjacent cells through their canaliculi. Questions involving bone resorption have persisted for years and have been mainly concerned with the role of the osteoclast in the process. Microscopic examinations lend strong support to the majority opinion that the larger multicellular (multilobulor) cell excretes a solvent which dissolves the inorganic salts while the organic matrix is digested by the cell itself. Recent studies indicate that this is an oversimplification.

Studies indicate that more than salts and matrix are involved in changes in bone. The ground substance, tissue fluid, and the balance of the blood elements prevailing at the time all contribute. This has been shown by Schour and Ham (1934), and Weinmann and Schour (1945). Both these studies revealed an elevation of blood, calcium, and phosphorus with the administration of parathyroid hormone accompanied by a hypocalcification of the hard tissues forming at the time. Lehman, Engel, and Laskin (1959) have implicated changes in the soluble citrate level in the resorptive process of bone. By studying the egg-laying cycle in the pigeon, they showed that when the shell is forming there is pronounced disaggregation of medullary bone, which is quicky restored when the shell is complete.

Evidence such as this suggests a tide of constituents flowing through the skeletal system susceptible to being mobilized or demobilized as needed. It also emphasizes the importance of bone as a reservoir for inorganic salts constantly being withdrawn and replenished in a continually renewing skeleton. In this light, the inorganic constituents of a bone would change from year to year.

The previously mentioned studies can only be illustrated by chemical methods at present, since they occur at such a rapid rate. The most graphic method, that of vital staining of bone, is limited due to loss of definition at high magnification. Only in the areas of slowly growing periosteal or endosteal compact bone are the dye lines sufficiently defined to permit interpretation. This method has been used to study the movement of teeth by orthodontic forces, and raises questions. Is a continuous or an intermittent force more effective in tooth movement? Where is the center of rotation located when the tooth is tipped? Is there evidence for bending of alveolar bone under orthodontic pressure? How do the pressure or tension areas of a tooth socket differ under conditions of orthodontic stress?

The answers to all these questions involve the tissue immediately surrounding the root of the tooth, the periodontal ligament. The orthodontist should have a thorough understanding of this structure.

Early in the investigations at the University of Illinois, it was found that madder would not be eaten by monkeys, the animal researchers desired to study. It was thus necessary to change from a method of feeding by mouth to an intraperitoneal injection. Madder was abandoned in favor of alizarine, which was commercially available. Many stains were used, each made by a different manufacturer, and trials revealed that the synthetic form was not always taken up by growing bone. Finally, "alizarine Red S" was found to answer all the requirements. Dosages were worked out on the basis of body weight of the experimental animal.

Schour, in 1934, had already demonstrated the incremental growth of the rat incisor using sodium fluoride injections, but there were drawbacks when the technique was applied to bone studies. While a line could easily be seen in the homogeneous dentin, due to differences in refraction, in bone the contrast was difficult to detect due to the looser organization of the tissue. Alizarine Red S met all the objectives, leaving a sharp clean line of brilliant red which stood out like stripes on a stick of peppermint candy when the specimen was sectioned. This stain made it possible to lay out the pattern of incremental growth of teeth and to demonstrate that the rhythm was governed by the gradients of locus, time, rate, and age. Indeed, Steadman demonstrated the resultant was an Archimedial spiral.

It was found that if more than a generalized surface study was desired the specimen had to be sectioned, the reason being the translucency of fresh bone tissue. If one is dealing with a flat bone which has been vitally stained, the color will appear to be on the surface even though there has been no injection for two or three weeks. On sectioning at right angles to the surface to be studied, a thick layer of clear bone will be found outside the stained bone. This was further demonstrated by Levine, in 1940, who placed implants of dental amalgam in the perietal bones of rabbits. On sacrifice at the end of the period of growth the amalgam plugs appeared bright and shiny, but it was impossible to place divider points in the measuring holes in the amalgam. Sectioning the bone at right angles to its surface, through the amalgam, revealed three or four lamellae of clear bone overlying the implant.

Massler, Schour, and Brodie undertook the study of cranial growth in the macaque monkey using a vital dye, since it had been taught that the brain case enlarged by deposition of bone on the outside and resorption within. Indeed, Brash denied any role to the sutures. Alizarine injections revealed that deposition took place on the *inner* surface of the inner table of bone, while sutural growth seemed to be pushing or pulling the bones apart. Thus enlargement of the cranium seemed to be a function of the sutures, while increase in thickness of the calvarium was a function of the internal surface. The stained lines of alizarine were found to come together in the region of the forehead just above the frontal sinuses, and from there down reappeared on the outside of the face. At first, growth of the face appeared generalized with the outer surfaces of the entire bones stained, but at the equivalent to the fourth or fifth human year the monkey staining became localized and there arose the tendency to speak of growth "centers." Such centers were probably the chief contributors to growth from the beginning, their relatively greater contribution being masked by the earlier generalized staining. See Fig. 22a.

Distrust in the use of alizarine stain in thin layers of bone such as the wall of the nose, floor, and wall of the orbit arose from Levine's studies in the rabbit. For this reason, an extension of Brash's study on the growth of the upper face in the pig was undertaken by Moore using the macaque monkey. Moore's problem was to devise a technique for examining sections of the whole head without decalcification, which of course would loosen the stain. The solution was to embed the head in a block of plastic and then face cut the block on a lathe. To provide a record, color photographs were taken on successive cuts until the whole skull had been examined in a medio-lateral direction.

Again, there was heavy stain showing on the sur-

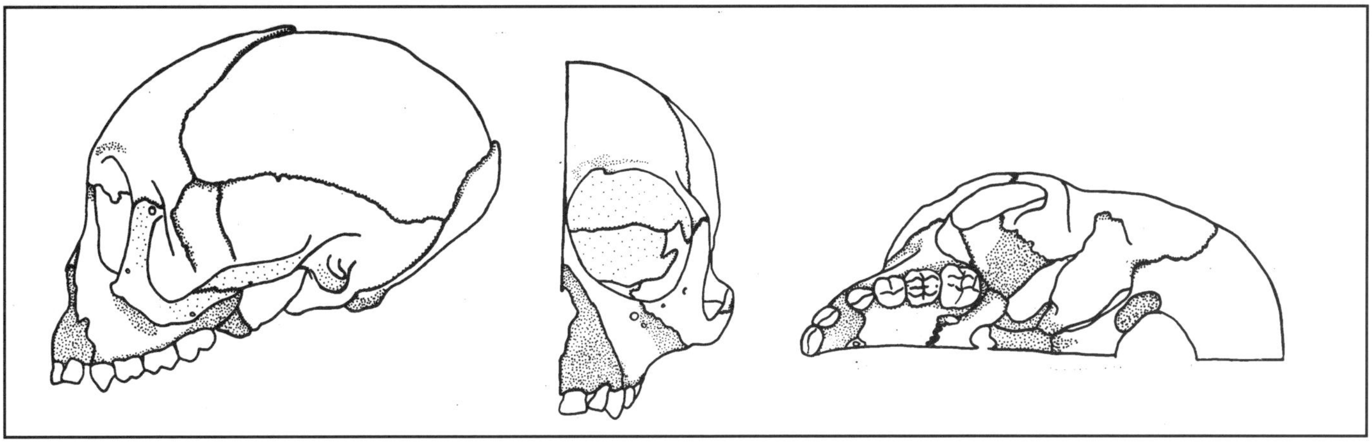

Fig. 22a.

face of the premaxilla, in the area of the second molar in the maxilla and the area adjacent to the pterygoid plate. There was slightly less stain at the junction of the maxilla at the zygomatic bone and at the frontal bone in the midline. Basal views of the monkey skull showed heavy staining on the surface of the body and great wing of the sphenoid and the occipital condyles. All together the localities of increased bone growth revealed by the alizarin indicated that the maxilla had moved downward and forward; there was more stain on the maxillary sides of the frontomaxillary and zygomaticomaxillary sutures. This forward movement seemed to be the result of prolific additions of bone laid down between the posterior surface of the maxilla and the pterygoid process. It could not fail to impress one with its similarity to the growth pattern of the mandible. It seemed active growth of the occipital condyle not only increased height of the head, but also maintained its proportion to vertical growth of the whole body.

Although alizarine continues to be widely employed for vital staining of bone, other agents have come into use, including purpurin and tetracyclines. All are employed in a similar manner and all require sacrifice of the experimental animal and the subsequent grinding of bone sections to distinguish markings of the agent. This is not only a tedious process, but also restricts the cutting of sections to relatively thick slices.

Okada and Nimura utilized lead acetate injections to demonstrate deposition lines on teeth. The lead was precipitated by sulphur dioxide during decalcification and sectioning by a microtome. Later, Zak wrote on the use of "lead acetate vital staining as a means of demonstrating bone growth patterns." See Fig. 22b. Although these methods eliminate wearisome grinding of sections, there still are disadvantages in the occasional loss or diffusion of materials during fixation and decalcification. More recent and sophisticated techniques for the application of vital dyes have been developed in Engel's laboratory.

Examining thin ground sections of bone, Enlow has explained how relocation of bony areas takes place. He explains how an area of cancellous bone at one stage of growth becomes compact bone at another stage and vice versa. Using similar methods he has shown how bone can be reshaped or redesigned. All such alterations occur as a result of additive or subtractive processes, and these can take place on any bony surface not covered by other bone.

Reading list:

Scheiman Tagger, Etty, and Brodie, Allan G. "Lead Acetate as a Marker of Growing Calcified Tissues. A Modified Method." *Anatomical Record,* 150, 1964. Press of the Wistar Institute of Anatomy and Biology, Philadelphia, PA.

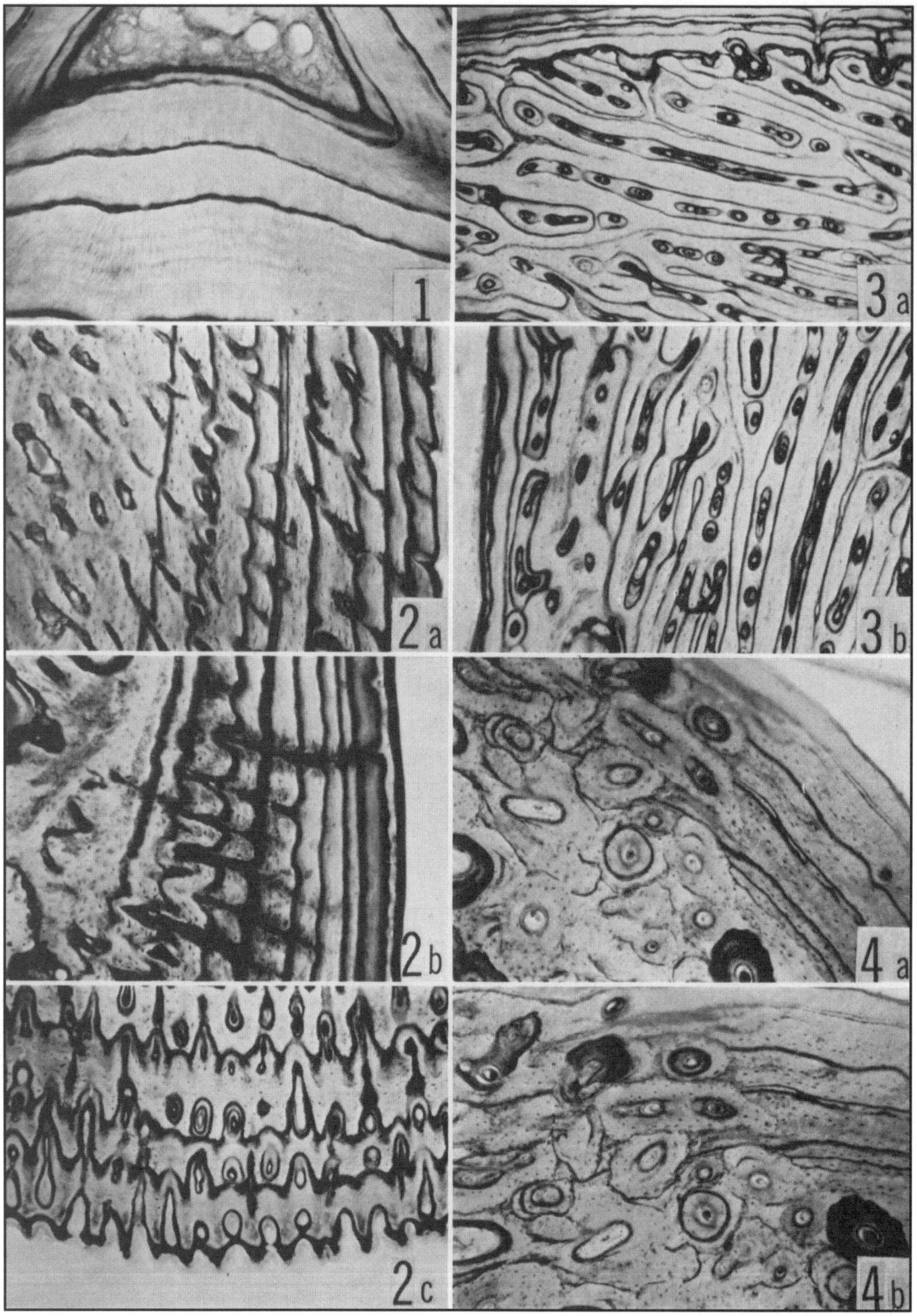

Fig. 22b.1: Cross section through mandibular incisor of a rabbit, the four lead lines contrasting with the much fainter contour lines of Owen. 2: Frontal section through the body of the rabbit's mandible; a: Middle portion—straight, closely spaced lines indicate relatively slow periosteal apposition on the lateral border; b: Transitional area from lateral to lower border of the mandible. This spacing gradually increases toward the lower border; c: Lower border—lanceolated lines and greater spacing indicate fast growth. 3: Longitudinal section of the shaft of the femur in a growing Rhesus monkey; a: Periosteal apposition and primary osteones, figure rotated 90 degrees counterclockwise; b: Endosteal apposition and primary osteones. 4: Cross section through the shaft of the femur of a growing rabbit; a and b: Bone remodeling, resulting in the formation of Haversian systems at the expense of circumferential lamellae. All stages of osteone formation can be observed.

23.
The Skeleton of the Head

Earlier we discussed the phylogeny of the head and pointed out that the beginning of movement on the part of early water living forms was probably the chief determinant of the vertebrate form of organization. This form was elongate and symmetrical and gave direction to movement. It was likewise in the interest of survival that the end organs of the special senses should be gathered at the forward end, since it would be upon these that the animal would depend to locate food and avoid enemies. The special senses would be the first parts to enter a new environment.

It should not be inferred that these organs or parts moved forward into places already prepared for them. As each evolved, it was supported or protected by specialized tissue around it so that the collection which ultimately formed the head in the beginning could be looked upon as a relatively loose collection of parts that were individually well advanced, but each was connected with the central nervous system.

The food and oxygen procuring mechanisms might be thought of as lying separated from the special sense organs. Both were served by a special group of bones which constituted jaws and which helped to form a stomodeum. The stomodeum acted as the portal or trap for both food and oxygen.

The impact of a totally different environment on those forms that emerged from water demanded sweeping adaptations. In air they had to resist gravity. This required firmer organization and greatly increased strength of their supporting framework. Both called for calcified skeletons in the place of cartilage and armor scales. But an even greater need was the demand for energy. Not only was movement essential but, if they were to free themselves of water entirely, they had to buffer themselves against the wide fluctuations of temperature that characterize a terrestrial existence. They had to become warm-blooded in order to maintain a higher and a stable level of metabolism.

Since energy enters the animal body as food and oxygen, the parts responsible for the gathering of these essentials were enormously increased in efficiency. Although teeth had already appeared, they were poorly attached. Now they became complex in design and were supported by bone to withstand the increased stresses put upon them. A loosely organized head skeleton would no longer serve as a foundation against which they could function, and this was likewise strengthened.

The gill arches could not supply sufficient oxygen to serve the increase in the food intake, and the respiratory system adapted accordingly. A slit had appeared in the ventral wall of the gut and this led into a closed pouch, capable of holding a small quantity of air. This pouch began to spread down inside the thoracic cage and to lobulate until it offered vast surface for the absorption of oxygen.

Accompanying this, a perforation appeared in back of the palate, in the dorsal wall of the gut. This provided an opening between what was to be the nose and the gut. This served olfaction admirably, since air flowing through the nasal pits passed over the olfactory lobes of the brain. At the same time it brought about a crossing of the food and air tracts at a lower level. This necessitated a valve to prevent both being open simultaneously. The larynx was, and still is, this valve.

It will be recalled that the early head was made up of a number of "sets" of bones, each apparently devoted to the protection and support of the special end organs. There was an internal complex serving similar functions for the brain. The gradual evolution to the modern head was a process which witnessed a reduction in the numbers of bones with an increase in complexity of the survivors (Williston's Law).

It is not known whether the process by which this came about was one of fusion of adjacent elements or of the dominance of one in a group that gradually pushed others into oblivion. There is evidence for both arguments. In either event the result was the same, viz., the 22 bones of the mammalian head. With few exceptions those surviving bones are complex in design, and each serves several functions. This brings us to a consideration of the several functions that bones serve.

When one thinks of the skeleton one is apt to

consider first its supportive function. It lends the rigidity to the body that permits it to resist the continuous pull of gravity. But this is the passive aspect; action or movement calls for greater strength, due the transmission of sudden shock as in walking or jumping.

Bones also act as levers to which muscles are attached and by their arrangement not only provide for the movements of the body but also for the maintenance of its posture. Movement represents muscles in temporary disequilibrium while the body at rest represents an equilibrium of antagonizing muscle forces. More will be said about this later.

In the case of the higher apes, and even more so in humans, bones have a protective function. This is the main function of the skullcap.

Finally, there are certain bones that have for their chief function the support of delicate membranes in the most effective positions to serve the functions for which they are intended. The turbinates of the nose are in this category. Light and spongy, they offer sufficient support to the nasal mucosa to maintain the channels of the upper airway and by their convolutions provide maximum surface for contact with the inspired air.

For the present purposes we are eliminating the roles that the bones play in hemopoiesis and in the storage of calcium and phosphorus. These functions do not enter into matters of design.

When man undertakes to create anything that has for its object the doing of work or the withstanding of stress, he directs his attention first to its design or form and second to the material from which he will fashion it. His experience has taught him that there are certain forms and certain qualities that best serve specific demands. Thus, if he wishes to suspend weight, passively, he is apt to use wires and cables since these have tensile strength and are most economical of material. If he wishes to support weight most economically, he employs a hollow pipe and an "I," "T," or "L" beam. Where it is necessary to provide or protect space beneath the weight, he makes use of arch or dome design.

But the general design is only a part of the solution. An equally important factor is the physical nature of the material he intends to use and the spatial arrangements of its constituents.

The wire or cable, for all of its strength and economy, would be worthless if stability of the suspended object were necessary. A steel hollow pipe would be necessary for a single supporting element where there were apt to be even light lateral forces working, while cast iron hollow pipes supporting arches or domes would serve equally well where such forces might be present. If domes or arches are subject to intermittent shock or strain they may be enormously strengthened by lamination, as exhibited in automobile springs or the long arches used to support roofs today.

One of the most striking examples of the utilization of design, combined with the arrangement of constituent elements, is seen in the crane. Evolving over the years from a tree trunk with a pulley at the end, it has come to represent a maximum of strength derived from a minimum of material. The crisscrossing of relatively light, short straps of metal connecting its main members provides alternating pathways of tensions and shearing forces that counteract each other, enabling the crane to sustain great weight, even at right angles to its axis.

In learning to use principles of design and to utilize materials, man had only applied or infringed the "basic patents" of nature, as Gregory so aptly put it. There is probably no place where this is so clearly shown as in the skeleton. A very nice analogy may be drawn between the paleontology of the head skeleton of man and the evolution of the gasoline engine in the automobile. Starting with an explosion chamber, it was quickly discovered that a cooling system was essential. This took the form of a copper and asbestos jacket, with water circulation through a radiator. Then came a lubricating system with jets supplying oil to each movable part. In the course of the circulation each of these was represented by a thin glass tube on the dashboard which showed the driver the condition of lubrication at each movable part. Then provision had to be made for ignition, which was furnished by a magneto activated by hand cranking. If the driver was caught out after dark he had to dismount, turn the acetylene tank on the running board over, and light the gas in each headlight.

The point that should be remembered here is that this early engine was an accumulation of systems, added one after the other as the demand arose. Each system was more or less complete unto itself and made up of its own parts. Today, thanks to the pressures of competition and economy, the automobile engine has been simplified in the number of its parts while the individual parts have become more complex in design as they came to serve more than one function. The engine block, for instance, now provides not only the explosion chamber but also contributes to the circulating system and the lubricating system while furnishing attachment for the starter, lights, etc. It is cast in a single block.

In a similar manner the bones of the head have been greatly reduced in number and increased in complexity. The maxilla, for instance, which was originally a simple trough-like scale on the margin of the stomodeum, has come to furnish a large part of the lateral wall of the nose, almost the entire floor of the orbit, the maxillary sinus, nearly three quarters of the hard palate, and the three main stress pathways of the face. It still carries the upper teeth, which seems to have been its original function, but in addition to this has come to make important contributions to such diverse functions as deglutition, respiration, sight, mastication, speech, and even to olfaction. Each of these functions places different demands upon it, demands that can be met efficiently with the greatest economy of substance only by the utmost refinement of design and strategic disposition of structural elements.

All of this adds up to something like the following as a Law of Bone Design: "A bone may be taken as representing the most efficient arrangement of the least amount of material to carry the peak of the load of its several functions."

I know that you all have had a course in human anatomy and probably in histology as well. I know further, from personal experience, that it was not particularly stimulating since it seemed to be largely the memorizing of a great number of details in which you were not particularly interested. But when anatomy is studied from the aspect of the reasons for these details, it becomes one of the most fascinating fields in biology. Unfortunately, it can be learned from this aspect only after one knows the facts and can build upon them. Without the foundation of facts it becomes a fascinating fairy study—and equally subject to suspicion.

Analysis of the Bones of the Head

In analyzing the individual bones of the head, it is extremely helpful to keep in mind the phylogeny of each, i.e., where and when it originated, what functions it has served, and how it has changed over the ages. In addition to this, the attempt should be made to examine each of its parts in relation to the function or functions that it serves in humans. In the following several sections, this is the plan that will be followed as we proceed from bone to bone. However, it will be worthwhile occasionally to depart from this plan to consider functional areas to which several bones may contribute. Indeed, we must begin in this manner since the head is made up of two major parts, viz., the brain case and the face.

The Brain Case

The brain case is composed of eight bones, viz., the occipital, sphenoid, ethmoid, frontal, two temporal, and two parietal. Articulated, they represent two structures of different functions. The inner surface, composed of compact bone, can be looked upon as a part serving the brain, with which it lies in close contact. It grows as long as the brain grows and stops when the brain stops, following the neural curve of growth.

Over this inner brain envelope is a second part that belongs to the skeletal system and largely follows its growth. This consists of extra layers, ridges, and buttresses which have for their function the sustaining of forces and the transmission of shocks which reach it from the body or from without. In some areas the inner and outer shells are separated either by spongy bone or by sinuses, and in others they unite to form a single layer of compact bone.

The Occipital Bone

The occipital bone (Fig. 23a) is made up of four parts, viz., the squama, the lateral masses, and the basilar part. From the beginning it has been the main linkage between head and body. Viewed from this aspect it is desirable to think of the area immediately surrounding the foramen magnum, induding the condyles, as one of the most primitive parts of the bone.

The margin or rim of the foramen is composed of compact bone and is quite sturdy. In some cases it is extended downward as a collar by a fusion with the posterior ring of the atlas. In these cases, movements of the head must take place between

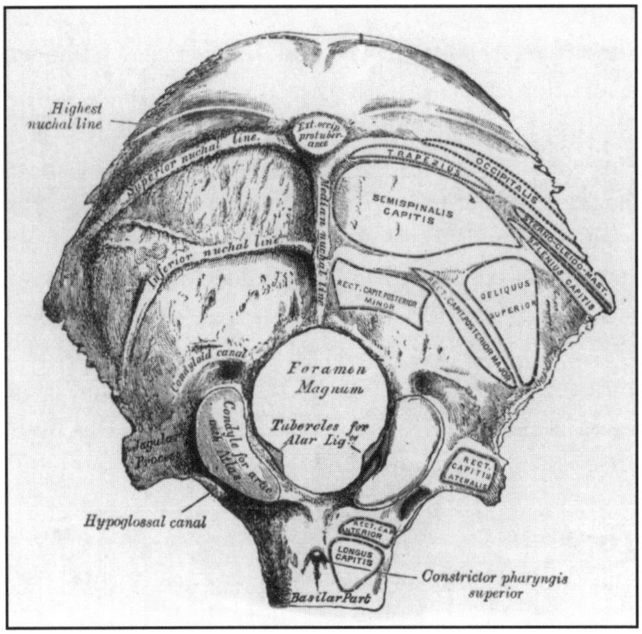

Fig. 23a. The occipital bone.

the atlas and the axis or epistropheus. Lying on either side of foramen magnum, and extending from near the middle of the lateral border to its anterior margin, are the occipital condyles. Their course is forward and medialward and their convex articular surfaces face downward, outward, and slightly forward. Their main support is derived from the basilar part of the bone, which lies anterior and medial to them.

Lateral to each condyle lies a heavy buttress of bone which terminates forward in a large scallop. This helps to form the jugular foramen in the articulated skull. Laterally and posteriorly to this notch is the jugular process, a heavy, quadrilateral buttress of bone which articulates with the like-named process of the petrous part of the temporal bone.

Continuous with the back of the lateral parts and completing the foramen magnum is the planum nuchale of the squama. In this area the inner and outer tables of the skull form a single layer of compact bone so thin that it will frequently transmit light in the dry state. The outer surface presents a midsagittal nuchal crest and two transverse crests, the superior and inferior nuchal lines. The area between these lines is roughened for attachment of the heavy postcervical muscles which hold the head erect. In four-footed animals the nuchal area of the bone is relatively larger than in humans and frequently ends above in a crest which affords additional attachment. In these horizontally oriented forms the head is placed forward of, instead of on top of, the vertebral column. Thus, great muscle tension is required to keep it from dropping.

At the middle of the squama is the external occipital protuberance, and flowing laterally from it are two crests, the superior and the highest nuchal lines. The protuberance may vary from a slight elevation to a pronounced process shaped like a hawk's beak. It, together with the middle nuchal line, gives attachment to the ligamentum nuchae, the check-rein of the head.

In back and above the nuchal area of the squama lies the planum occipitale, a smooth-domed area that extends to the lambdoidal suture where it joins the parietal bones. It is covered by a dense, tough connective tissue, the galea aponeurotica. This part of the squama, lying above the superior nuchal lines, reveals a structure that is in marked contrast to the nuchal area. Now the bone abruptly becomes three-layered with outer and inner layers of compact bone, separated by diploe.

The planum occipitale, while not exclusively a human characteristic, is nearly so. In all animals below the great apes, the brain case is covered by the temporalis muscle. With the great expansion of the brain and the resulting increase in size of its case, the muscles of posture and of mastication were left behind. The bones covering the top of the brain were exposed to trauma from above. The adaptive response to this critical need was the dome-shaped head of humans, further strengthened and made resistant to sharp blows by a lamination of its layers. As we shall see as we proceed in these lectures, this protective arrangement is carried forward the entire extent of the head to the supra-orbital margins of the frontal bone and extends down the sides of the cranium to the place where the temporalis muscle affords protection.

The basilar part of the occipital bone lies anterior to the foramen magnum. Its superior and inferior surfaces are quadrilateral, but in profile it is seen to be triangular with its apex directed downward and backward. This apex represents the anthropological point "basion," which is taken as the midpoint of the anterior border of foramen magnum. A strong ligament connects this area with the dens of the epistropheus and serves to make this the point of least movement between the head and body. The base of the triangle faces forward and upward and meets a like surface, the back of the sphenoidal body. A plate of cartilage separates the two in early life, and the junction is known as the spheno-occipital synchondrosis.

A section of the basilar part reveals that it is completely enclosed by compact bone. Its core is cancellous or may be partially and completely hollowed out by the invasion of the sphenoidal sinus with growth. When the occipital bone is oriented in its usual manner in the living and viewed from the side, the significance of the design and structure of the basilar part becomes apparent.

Remembering that the condyles rest on the top of the vertebral column, it can be seen that all stresses and shocks reaching the head from the body (running or jumping) must enter the head here. Since force travels in a straight line, these shocks would be conveyed to the brain were it not for the strengthening of structures around foramen magnum. Equally true is the fact that a force from below, meeting the convex surfaces of occipital condyles, would tend to be dissipated radially. But lying around the condyles and close to them are portals of entry and exit for vitally important structures, e.g., the foramen magnum itself, the jugular foramen, etc. Forces transmitted by the condyles are carried over pathways which lie between these portals.

Owing to the bilateral disposition of the condyles, their position toward the anterior part of the foramen magnum, and the forward and upward placement of the basilar part of the occipital bone, the major pathway for these stresses is medially, forward and upward. Thus, the significance of the pipe-like structure of the basilar element becomes obvious. This is the main stress pathway of the skull. Nor does it share its load with the bones on either side of it, the petrous element of the temporals. To these it is connected by fibrous tissue alone, and even this tenous connection is broken by the large jugular foramen.

Forming the posterolateral boundary of the jugular foramen is another buttress, the jugular process, the form of structure of which is similar to the basilar part. It too is of hollow pipe design, and it is likewise separated by a plate of cartilage from articulation with the temporal. Its articulating surface faces laterally and very slightly forward so that the forces it receives from the condyles are transmitted in that direction. Light vectors of force that might have a backward, or backward and lateral, direction are carried around the foramen magnum to the middle nuchal line or dissipated through the heavy bone lying posterior to the temporalis muscle.

If you have wondered why so much time has been devoted to the occipital bone, a bone that is not usually considered of dental interest, it is because it exemplifies so clearly certain principles of adaptations to functions, adaptations that are more difficult to discern in other parts of the head skeleton. Let us briefly summarize these.

Each part of the occipital bone serves different functions. The internal table of the squama of the bone serves the purpose of containing and supporting the brain. A delicate jelly dish would serve equally well and the planum nuchale does just this. The external surface is divided into two distinct parts. The nuchal part is roughened for the attachment of some of the great muscles of the neck, strengthened only by a few reinforcing ribs to carry small, posteriorly directed forces and to protect this fragile area against torsion. It is thoroughly protected from direct forces from without by its massive muscular covering.

The planum occipitale, on the contrary, reveals the increasing need for protection from above as the brain and its case expanded. Here, both the form and three-layered structure are perfect adaptations for protection.

The condyles, withstanding all stresses coming from the body, are given the necessary support to resist them by buttresses which immediately transmit all such stresses away from vital parts. They represent the areas of least movement between head and body. It is a general principle that nerves and blood vessels enter all bones near their centers of least movement, but nowhere in the body is this more critical than around the foramen magnum. Here are found not only the brain stem but also all of the major blood channels of the head with the exception of the carotid artery. We shall see later how this is protected.

The Sphenoid Bone

The sphenoid bone forms an important part of the base of the cranium and is situated in the midline, anterior to the basilar part of the occipital bone. It consists of a body, two great wings, two

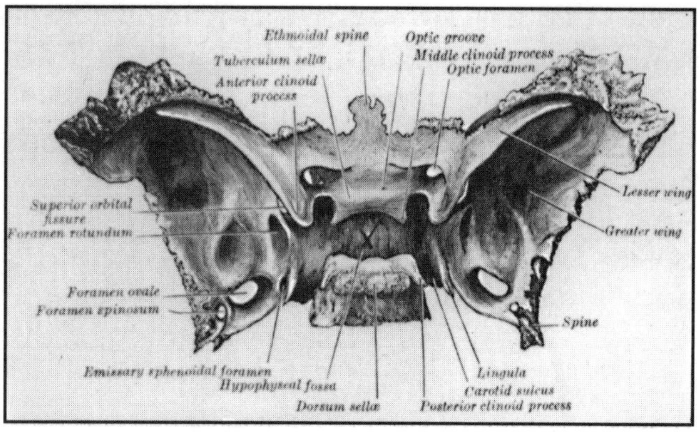

Fig. 23b. The sphenoid bone.

small wings, and two pterygoid processes (Fig. 23b). Because of its numerous landmarks, this bone is a nightmare for the student. Indeed, it is told of Oliver Wendell Holmes, when he was professor of anatomy at Harvard, that he would hold this bone up before his class and begin his lecture with, "Gentlemen, this is the sphenoid bone—damn the sphenoid bone." You probably shared this sentiment as students of anatomy. For the purpose of these lectures, however, it will not be necessary for us to engage in feats of memory. Our interest will be directed toward design of this bone as a force transmitter. We shall consider only those details that will serve to orient us in later studies of growth and of function.

The body of the sphenoid may be thought of as cuboidal in shape, separated until late childhood from the basilar part of the occipital by a plate of cartilage. Thus it continues the midline pillar forward and transmits the forces travelling in this direction from the occipital condyles. Its structure is similar to that of the basi-occipital, being composed of spongiosa surrounded by compact bone in early life. The spongiosa is gradually eliminated by invasion from the posterior, superior part of the nasal cavity resulting in the sphenoidal sinuses. Following the elimination of the synchondrosis and the union of the sphenoid and occipital bones, the sinuses may extend into the basi-occipital.

The strong midline pillar ends abruptly at the end of the anterior surface of the sphenoid body. Here we find superiorly a thin horizontal ridge, a midsagittal crest, and two lateral margins which articulate with the cribriform plate of the ethmoid and orbital roofs, the perpendicular plate of ethmoid, and the back of the ethmoidal labyrinth, respectively. These all are delicate structures, incapable of withstanding stress. Where then does then stress go?

From either side of the body the great wings extend laterally and forward forming most of the floor of the middle cranial fossa. Anteriorly and medially this surface curves backward and ends in a smooth margin, as the inferior boundary of the superior orbital fissure. More laterally it curves until it faces medially, and here it extends to a higher level. This surface constitutes the sphenoid's contribution to the inner wall of the brain case.

Another surface is completely on the outside of the skull. Its posterior margin is the same as that of the inner surface. Before the appearance of such landmarks as the infratemporal crest, i.e., in the young child, the superior and inferior surfaces of the great wing in this area tend to be parallel, but as age advances and external cranial landmarks become more prominent, the external or inferior surfaces flatten. Since the superior surface remains concave, an area of increasing thickness develops between them laterally. This lateral margin of the great wing forms a butt joint type of articulation with the squama of the temporal bone which is thought to be a site of lateral head growth during fetal and early postnatal life.

At the infratemporal line the external surface changes its direction rather abruptly and again follows a parallel course with the cranial surface, forming a part of the medial wall of the temporal fossa as it runs upward. We now approach the part of the great wing most difficult to visualize and the part upon which textbooks comment only briefly.

As the anterior margin of the vertical part of the great wing is approached there is again a separation of the outer and inner tables. The outer follows the concave wall of the temporal fossa, the inner the concave anterior wall of the middle cranial fossa. The resulting smooth area between them constitutes the lateral wall of the orbit. Thus, it may be seen that these three surfaces result from the meeting of three soft tissue masses, viz., the middle lobe of the brain, the eyeball, and the bulk of the temporalis muscle.

Now three surfaces which meet in this manner require a fourth surface to complete a pyramid, which the tip of the great wing is said to be. This fourth surface is entirely articular and is the one in which we are particularly interested because it is an essential part of the stress-bearing system of the head.

If the disarticulated frontal bone is viewed from below, there will be seen two roughened articular surfaces at the sides and toward the back of the smooth orbital plates. These areas extend upward and laterally on the frontal bone and receive the articular surface of the sphenoid wing just described. We shall reserve comment on this until we have considered the frontal bone.

The final parts of the sphenoid bone to engage our attention are the pterygoid processes. These paired structures descend from the great wings at their junctions with the body. Each consists of two lamina or plates separated below by a triangular notch which receives the pyramidal process of the palatine bone. The medial plate forms the most posterior part of the lateral wall of the nose and is concerned with the functions of respiration, deglutition, olfaction, and speech. The lateral plate is concerned almost wholly with movements of the mandible, affording origin for both the internal and external pterygoid muscles. The pterygoid processes also are concerned with a stress system of the face, as we shall see.

The Frontal Bone

The frontal bone (Fig. 23c) is another example of a single skeletal unit serving a number of functions. It usually is described as consisting of two parts: the squama and the orbital plates. As we shall see, the number of functions that this bone serves belies this apparent simplicity.

The squama or vertical part forms the entire forehead and a considerable part of the side of the skull. Viewing it from within, it is seen to be concave everywhere. This surface is in intimate contact with the surfaces of the hemispheres of the forebrain. Thc floor of the anterior cranial fossa is formed by the two thin orbital plates which bulge faintly upward and reflect the juxtaposition of the orbital contents and the inferior surface of the forebrain. The two orbital plates are separated by a notch which receives the cribriform plate of the ethinoid bone. This will be considered with the facial skeleton.

The inner plate of the squama is of compact bone and is overlaid by another and heavier cover-

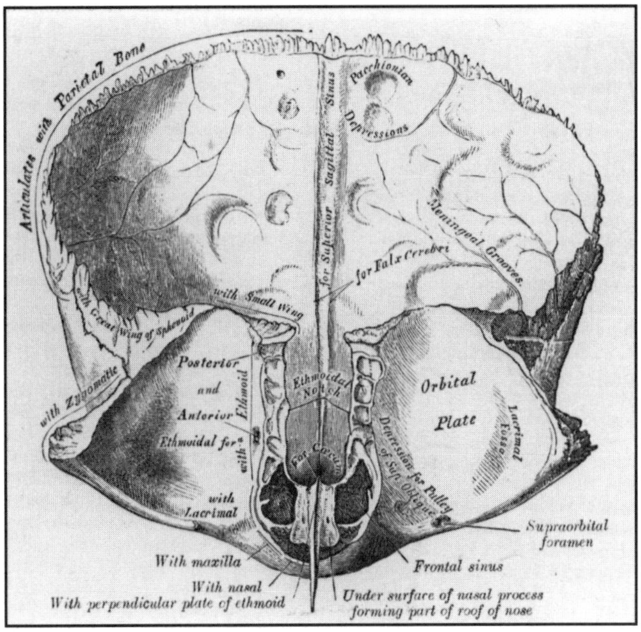

Fig. 23c. The frontal bone.

ing of compact bone from which it is separated by diploe throughout much of its extent. It exhibits, in short, the same architectural arrangement that was seen in the exposed part of the occipital squama. As was the case in the occipital area, the frontal squama is exposed and the domed, laminated structure is admirably designed to withstand blows from above.

Midway down the squama, just below the frontal prominences, the inner and outer plates diverge from each other at about the fourth to sixth year and the diploe increases. Somewhat later an invasion of this diploe takes place, this time from the upper anterior part of the nose. This, the frontal sinus, extends to various limits between the tables, both superiorly and laterally. In some individuals, principally males, the supra-orbital ridges are extremely prominent and the sinuses extend laterally to the zygomatic processes. However, this prominence is not a reliable guide to the size of the sinuses as a complete absence of sinus is not infrequently demonstrated by the x-ray.

Midsagittaly a thin bony spine projects downward and forward between the openings of the right and left sinuses. This is the frontal spine which lends support to the two nasal bones. When one views the disarticulated bone from below and in front, the bilateral sinus openings reveal the wide separation between the inner and outer tables. The outer, free table receives the nasal bones medially and the frontonasal processes of the maxilla laterally. This entire articular area of the external table is known as the nasal notch and its highest midline point is the anthropologic point Nasion. Laterally from the nasal notch, the junction of the squama and the orbital plate forms the supra-orbital margin. Beginning as a rounded continuation of the side of the bridge of the nose, it becomes progressively sharper until it ends in the zygomatic process.

The zygomatic process is a strong buttress of bone located at the junction of the vertical, orbital, and temporal surfaces of the bone as though the external table had been pulled laterally and forward to provide legs for the support of the frontal bone. And this is exactly the function of these pillars. As we shall see, they are part of the stress pathways which carry the forces of occlusion.

Back of the zygomatic process lies the triangular area that receives the articular surface of the sphenoid wing. The most inferior margin of this area can be seen near the top of the lateral wall of the orbit. From this margin the articular surface extends upward and laterally following the concavity of the inner table. In this manner the great wings of the sphenoid come to embrace and support the globular frontal. The limit of this junction, shown by a suture line, can be seen in the temporal fossa at a considerably higher level than that in the orbit.

The Parietal Bone

The parietal bones form the domed bridge between the frontal and occipital squamas. They are the simplest in design of any of the head bones and their functions can be easily interpreted. Their inner surfaces protect the brain and complete its housing above. They are everywhere laminated through dense inner and outer layers separated by diploe. They protect the brain against blows from above.

The sutures which constitute their borders are of interest to us because of their implied relation to the growth of the brain. At their meeting above in the midsagittal plane they are denticulated so that they could allow limited hinge movement without pulling apart as the base of the brain expanded. Anteriorly they meet the posterior edge of the frontal squama in a double bevel, lapping this bone above and being lapped by it on the side.

The posterior edges are heavily denticulated where they meet the occipital squama while the inferior margin in back articulates with the mastoid process of the temporal and with the squama of the same bone anteriorly. This last area presents a large notch and is strongly bevelled at the expense of its outer table. The bevelled articular area is only faintly marked, indicating a weak articulation.

The Temporal Bone

The temporal bone (Fig. 23d) lies at the side and base of the skull and closes the interval between the occipital, sphenoid, and parietal bones. It is described as having four main parts, viz., squama, mastoid, petrous, and tympanic parts, all of which can be discerned as separate entities in the x-ray taken at birth.

The squama of the bone, thin and translucent, is the most superior part of the bone and is a part of the brain case proper. The superior margin of the squama is markedly convex, forming an arc of 180° and bevelled throughout much of its course at the expense of its inner surface throughout the posterior two-thirds of its extent. This bevel laps the like surface of the inferior margin of the parietal bone referred to in the description of that bone. Anterior to this it laps the posterior margin of the great wing.

A faint curved ridge, the temporal line, extends downward and forward from the junction between the squama and the mastoid parts and passes above

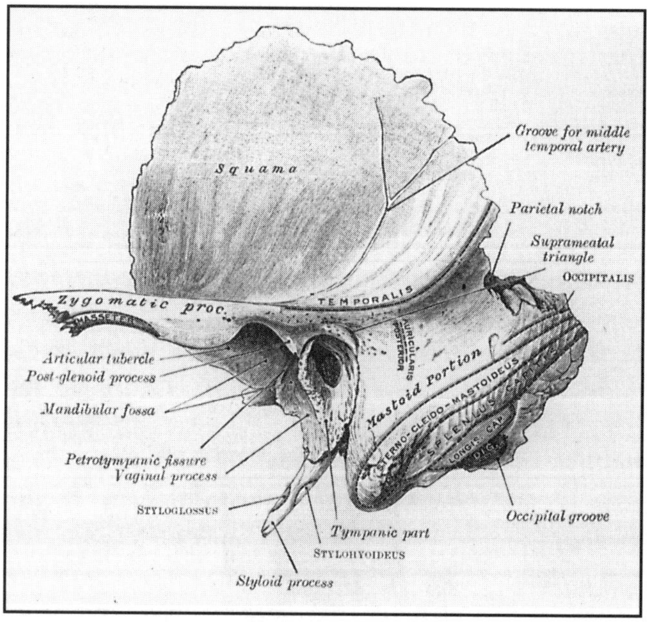

Fig 23d. The temporal bone.

the external ear opening. Here it becomes horizontal and, diverging from the side of the skull and then running forward, it becomes the superior edge of the zygomatic process.

Anteriorly and below, at the level of the inferior border of the zygomatic process, the external surface of the squama bends medially to form part of the base of the skull. The junction of the two surfaces constitutes a continuation of the infratemporal crest, which was discussed with the great wing of the sphenoid.

The posterior border of this inferior surface of the squama forms the anterior boundary of the glenoid fossa, a depression of varying depth which receives the condyle of the mandible. From the junction of the temporal and infratemporal surfaces with the anterior wall of the fossa arises the anterior root of the zygomatic process. This root, in contrast to the posterior root, is sturdy. It projects laterally from the bone and the lateral half of its inferior surface is known as the articular eminence. It will be considered in greater detail with the temporomandibular joint.

The roof of the glenoid fossa is separated from the brain case only by a thin plate of bone. From here it arches downward posteriorly to end as the anterior margin of the petrotympanic or Glaserian fissure. At about the middle of this border a small bony projection can be seen: the postglenoid process. Poorly developed in humans, it is very prominent in carnivorous animals, acting to prevent retrusion of the mandible. The area behind the Glaserian fissure is the nonarticular part of the glenoid fossa. It houses the tip of the parotid gland and is formed by the tympanic part of the bone.

The tympanic part appears to be wedged between the squama in front and the mastoid and petrous parts in back. The thin plate of bone that forms the back wall of the glenoid fossa also forms the anterior wall of the bony ear canal. This surface curves backward and then upward so that it forms the floor and part of the posterior wall of the canal. The roof and upper posterior wall are formed by the squama at its junction with the mastoid part.

Posteriorly, the tympanic part blends with the squama and mastoid part. Anteriorly and laterally as we have seen it forms the posterior border of the petrotympanic fissure while it fuses with the petrous part medially. The medial part of the lower border is thin. It splits laterally to enclose the root of the styloid process.

The mastoid part lies behind the tympanic part and below and somewhat in back of the squama, from which it is separated by the parietal notch. The articulation of this part of the bone with the parietal is a firm one, as shown by the extent of its surface and its heavy denticulations. Below this, and on the base of the skull, the mastoid part is similarly attached to the occipital.

The mastoid process itself is a large roughened projection which extends downward to varying degrees. It is especially prominent in the male. It is sometimes found to be filled with diploe and at other times to be almost completely pneumatized. Our chief interest in it lies in the fact that it is the most laterally disposed part of the head for muscle insertions, giving attachment to the sternocleidomastoid muscle. On the medial side of its base is a groove which affords origin to the posterior belly of the digastric muscle. The only landmark on the inside or cranial surface of the mastoid part is a large grooved channel for the housing of the sigmoid sinus.

The petrous part of the temporal bone is pyramidal in shape extending medially, forward and very slightly upward. Its base is fused with the inner surfaces of the squama and the mastoid part. Its apex is received in the angular interval between the basilar part of the occipital bone and the posterior margin of the great wing of the sphenoid. The pyramid has three surfaces and three borders, but for the purposes of these lectures it will be unnecessary to consider more than a few of the many landmarks these present for examination.

The longest and sharpest border separates the middle and posterior fossae of the skull. It extends for the most lateral limits of these cavities almost to the base of the posterior clinoid process of sphenoidal body. Near its medial end it is notched for the ganglion of the trigeminal nerve.

It is important to note that the petrous part of the temporal bone is almost completely free of bony articulation with other bones. If one starts at the posterior lateral angle of the great wing of the sphenoid and follows the boundary of the angular interval into which the petrous pyramid fits, it is found that at no point is there bone-to-bone contact.

The connection between the anterior border of the pyramid and the posterior margin of the great wing is one of connective tissue which simultaneously holds the eustachian tube in place on the under surface of the skull. The tip of the petrous part is truncated and presents a large opening: the internal opening of the carotid canal. As a result a large opening, the foramen lacerum, exists, permitting communication between the inside and outside of the skull.

From the foramen lacerum backward, the tip of the petrous pyramid is connected to the basilar part of the occipital bone by fibrous tissue which on the superior side enters into the formation of the inferior petrosal sinus. In back of and lateral to this area the posterior border of the petrous pyramid is deeply notched for the reception of the jugular bulb. Only lateral to this does bony contact occur through the articulation of the jugular process.

From all that has been said about the temporal bone and its relation to other bones of the cranium, it can be seen that it is admirably protected against shock and stress. In back it is firmly united with the occipital bone and the posterior inferior angle of the parietal. The extensive lapping of the squama, parietal, and sphenoid wing acts as a zone of adjustment during growth, and certain studies seem to indicate that the temporal bone retains its position in space while all of the rest of the head skeleton rotates around it.

Starting in late embryonic life the head begins a rotation that carries it from a position in which the eyes face downward to one in which they face forward. This is more than a mere rotation on the occipital condyles. The forebrain stops growing at about three years, but the hind brain continues. Indeed, the occipital part of the head skeleton continues to travel downward and backward until the early 20s.

We have noted the firm union of the occipital bone with the parietals, and this movement of the occipital would tend to draw these covering bones with it. Adjustment for this growth is made at the suture between the anterior margins of the parietals and posterior of the frontal bone. This, the coronal suture, is a double-bevelled joint, and late activity in the suture has been shown by vital staining.

The transmission of any shock emanating from the occipital condyles or from the top of the head is prevented from entering the petrous part of the bone by a complete absence of bone-to-bone contact, as we have seen. Thus, the organs of hearing and of equilibrium are well-protected.

The squama of the temporal bone, thin to the point of translucency, would appear to be the most vulnerable part of the bone. Here, however, is found the same condition that prevails over the nuchal area of the occipital bone. These areas are covered with a protective shield of musculature, and bone tissue has been reduced to a minimum. The only stress-resisting structure associated with the temporal bone is the zygomatic arch, which will be considered with the face.

When the area around the foramen magnum is studied, another fundamental principle can be clearly seen, viz., that blood supply and drainage, together with nerves, enter and leave movable parts of the skeleton as close as possible to the centers of least movement of the parts. Obviously, the foramen magnum itself, transmitting the medulla oblongata and its associated membranes and vessels, is most favorably situated, lying as it does between the condyles—the centers of all head movement. Immediately lateral to the condyle lies the jugular fossa, the bony housing of the jugular bulb which receives the venous drainage of the transverse and petrosal sinuses.

Arterial supply to the brain is likewise well-protected. The carotid canal, entering a large foramen in the inferior surface of the petrous part of the temporal bone, is turned at right angles to run forward and medialward. It is entirely enclosed within bone until it reaches the apex of the pyramid from which it emerges in the foramen lacerum at the posterior lateral angle of the body of the sphenoid.

The vertebral artery is similarly protected. Ascending the neck through the foramina of the upper six cervical vertebrae, it must travel laterally to pass through that of the atlas which is the most laterally disposed. From here it doubles back to wind behind the superior facet of the atlas and enters the skull through the foramen magnum, where it unites with its fellow of the opposite side to form the basilar artery. Thus, the blood flow through both of these vital arteries is insured against pinching by the same type of device that is seen in the service station where the air hose runs through a metal pipe when its direction must be changed, or in the laboratory where the hose to the bunsen burner may be wrapped with a coiled wire.

Reading list:

Alexander, R.M. *Bones—The Unity of Form and Function.* New York: Macmillan Publishing Co., 1994.

Enlow, Donald. *The Human Face.* New York: Hoeber Publishers, 1968.

Keith, Arthur. *Menders of the Maimed.* London: Oxford University Press, 1919.

24.
The Facial Skeleton

The Ethmoid Bone

Although the ethmoid is generally considered as a bone of the cranium, we shall consider it with the facial skeleton for reasons to be seen later.

The bone consists of four main parts, viz., the cribriform plate, the perpendicular plate, and the two lateral masses or labyrinths. For ease of comprehension it may be thought of as having the form of a "T" when viewed from in front, the lateral masses hanging from the ends of the cross member.

The horizontal and cribriform plate occupies the notch between the orbital plates of the frontal bone. The medial edges of the inferior surfaces of these plates present half air cells which are closed by like half cells on the superior aspect of the labyrinths. The cribriform plate supports the olfactory area of the brain, and its inferior surface forms the bony roof of the nasal cavity. This partition is perforated by numbers of foramina of transmission of the olfactory filaments.

Descending from the middle of the cribriform plate sagitally is the perpendicular plate, which forms the upper part of the bony nasal septum. In addition to the superior border which is fused to the cribriform plate, it has four margins which form a pentagonally-shaped plate. The anterior superior margin articulates above with the back of the nasal spine and with the crests of the two nasal bones below. The superior posterior margin articulates with the ethmoidal crest which runs down the middle of the anterior surface of the body of sphenoid. The posterior inferior margin runs downward and forward and articulates with the alae of the vomer. At the end of this articulation, the margin travels upward and forward to join the anterior superior margin. This last margin supports the cartilaginous septum of the nose.

The labyrinth or lateral masses lie between the nasal and orbital cavities. They may be thought of as accumulations of various sized air cells enclosed by delicate plates of bone for the most part. The medial plate forms the upper half of the lateral wall of the nose and carries the middle and superior concha. These are scrolls of delicate bony tissue which support the nasal membranes.

The lateral plate, or lamina papyracea, can be seen as it forms the major part of the medial wall of the orbit. In back it articulates with the lateral extremity of the anterior surface of the body of the sphenoid. Anteriorly it is deficient, and the air cells are closed by the lacrimal bone and more anteriorly by the frontonasal process of the maxilla.

The Maxilla

A detailed description of the maxilla hardly seems necessary for an audience of dental professionals and students, but there are certain aspects of this bone that are extremely important in connection with the matters we are discussing. These are given scant attention in anatomy texts.

You may recall from our considerations of the phylogenetic development of this bone that it first made its appearance as a bony sheath at the margin of the upper jaw. A number of like bones lay above and in back of it, separating it from those which housed the brain. Its gradual evolution to its present dominant position in the face is thought to be due to the fact that teeth first appeared on this bone. As these increased in size, complexity, and function, the maxilla and mandible likewise increased in strength and extended further and further toward the brain case.

By the time the mammalian stage was reached, the mandible had made contact with the temporal bone and the maxilla had pushed the nasal and lacrimal bones out of the way to make contact with the frontal and had established a firm relation with the zygomatic arch.

During the period of evolutionary development, the maxilla invaded areas formerly occupied by other bones and took over the function formerly served by them. In humans, its intricate design and structure reflects its adaptation to these additional functions. Besides mastication, it now contributes to respiration, deglutition, sight, olfaction, and speech, and each of these has left its mark on the architecture of the bone.

Considered as a skeletal unit the maxilla may be thought of as a large air cell, the maxillary sinus, the surfaces of which form two exterior faces and the walls of three cavities, viz., the mouth, the nose, and the orbit. This hollow pyramid is connected firmly to the head at only three points. Near the midline above it meets the outer table of the frontal bone; in back it rests against the pterygoid process and palatine bone, and laterally it is supported by the zygomas. At all other locations it is either completely free, as at the inferior orbital fissure and pterygopalatine fossa, or connected by means of extremely delicate edges, as at the medial edge of the orbital floor where it meets the lamina papyracea of the ethmoid.

The Bony Nose

We have now arrived at a point where we can begin to analyze what has been described and point out the adaptation which permits this bone to serve so many functions. One of the most important of these is respiration, but this means much more than providing a passageway for air.

The nose and accessory sinuses constitute an air conditioning unit developed by nature ages before humans thought of it. Furthermore, it embodies the same principles that have been found indispensable in the manufactured product. What are these principles?

I. Just as human engineers provide heating or cooling systems with enormous surface areas for the rapid absorption or dispersion of heat, so the nose provides, though its conchae, meatuses, and septum, large surfaces for warming the inspired air.

II. Just as the human engineer places baffle plates in a gas furnace to direct the flame from the burner to the inner wall of the fire chamber, so the conchae, by their forms and disposition, interrupt the air column and direct it to warm surfaces.

III. Since the length of time during which the air remains in contact with such surfaces determines the degree of heat that will be transferred, the velocity of the air has a direct bearing on the effectiveness of the exchange. In the nose this is provided for by a small nostril through which the air flows at considerable speed. It then enters the nasal chamber, which is of much larger size by comparison. The pressure falls and velocity diminishes. Then passing from the chamber, it gains velocity as it travels through the relatively small posterior choanae. But even this is not the full extent of the control over the speed of the air column.

The membranes of the nose are erectile tissue controlled by temperature. Under ordinary circumstances, i.e., when the surrounding air is about the same as the body temperature, this membranous covering hugs the bony surfaces to which it is attached. A frontal x-ray taken at such a time reveals the air passages free and open. However, a drop in temperature brings striking changes. Now the air passages appear cloudy. The membranes have swollen and the air stream is slowed.

Many have had the experience of going outdoors into a temperature of 10 to 20 degrees below zero F. Almost immediately, you experience the sensation of having a thin icicle in each nostril. What you are feeling is the contact of different areas of swollen membranes. Under such conditions any vigorous physical exertion cannot be continued for long because the reduced temperature of the inspired air prevents sufficient exchange of oxygen in the lungs.

IV. The next principle of the air conditioner that has been brought to a high state of effectiveness is insulation. It can readily be seen that the surfaces supplying heat to the air stream would lose temperature by the exchange. This is minimized by the most effective type of insulation, viz., dead air spaces. Consider that the nose enjoys the benefit of such cavities underneath from the mouth, above from the brain case, anteriorly and above from the frontal sinuses, above and behind from the sphenoidal sinuses, and on both sides from the ethmoidal air cells and orbits above and the maxillary sinuses below.

Thus it may be realized how importantly the area of the middle face serves that most vital function, respiration. But this function requires that the structures serving the air conditioning aspects of breathing be extremely light and delicate. At the same time, this same area must carry some of the heaviest shocks and loads of the body—those of mastication. To perform these two very different functions, further adaptations have been necessary. Let us see what they are.

I do not have to point out to you the location and form of the alveolar arch and its contained teeth. Together they constitute the widest part of the maxillae. They are thus peripheral to the respiratory area. Further than this, the bone which supports them is of the compact type and forms the facial and infratemporal aspect of the bone. Connecting the two sides of the arch is the hard palate, a vault of considerable strength and thickness. This is further strengthened by the nasal septum.

Directly above the roots of the principal chewing tooth of this jaw, the first permanent molar, the heavy outer table of the maxilla appears to have been pulled laterally to form what is called the jugal process. Its superior, posterior surface is articular and of considerable extent. It meets and is supported by the maxillary process of the zygomatic bone, which is undoubtedly the chief stress bearer of mastication.

As was mentioned earlier, there are two other points of support of the maxilla. One of these is the frontonasal process near the midline in front, and the other at the posterior end of the alveolar process. Note that both of these are associated with the outer table of the bone.

Turning now to the teeth, we find modifications of even these structures in conformity with the adaptations thus far noted. One of the first things that strikes us is the marked differences in design between the teeth of the upper and lower jaws. Why should upper molars have three roots, and the lower two? Why should the roots of upper teeth have considerably more surface area than those of the lower? Upper and lower teeth must carry the same load, must withstand the same shocks, since action and reaction are equal and opposite.

It is well known that teeth resist the forces put upon them by a tensing of the periodontal fibres. It requires no demonstration to realize that more fibres can be attached as surface is increased. The maxillary teeth must have more surface, because the forces they transmit through their fibers to their supporting bone must be distributed over a greater area because of the light, spongy nature of maxillary bone. Further than this, the forces must be directed over definite pathways capable of carrying them. The prime example of this is the distribution of the roots of maxillary molars. The major root is the palatal, which follows the course of the hard palate, while the buccal roots are embraced by the outside compact table. Thus they straddle the maxillary sinus which, in some individuals, extends downward almost to the bifurcation of the roots. So the surprising conclusion is reached that the teeth of the upper and lower jaws are different because we warm our air after breathing it! Reptiles, although air breathers, do not do this. They have remained cold-blooded, and the teeth of the two jaws do not show root modification.

The Zygomatic Bone

Like many of the bones we have considered, the zygomatic is the sole survivor of a series of scale-like bones which formerly covered the middle of the side of the head. Perforations took place in this shield, above and below the area now occupied by the zygomatic arch, resulting in the uncovering of the external muscles of mastication and the ultimate formation of the temporal and infratemporal fossae. The zygomatic bone since earliest times has been intimately associated with the movements of the jaw.

In all mammals the zygomatic arch, of which the zygoma is the major part, forms a flying buttress between the brain case in back and face in front. In many there is no bony connection between the mid-zygoma and the brain case; in some there is a postorbital bar and in others, as in the monkeys and humans, the postorbital bar becomes the frontosphenoidal process and affords complete bony housing for the eye. When this occurs, there is a union of the two main stress pathways of the head through the medium of the great wing of the sphenoid.

25.
Introduction to Skeletal Studies

Prior to the analysis of the skeleton, it seems appropriate to indicate the nature of the studies from which present concepts have been derived. Foremost among these was the observation that the form of a bone reflected its function. This concept is at least as old as Greek medicine, and was probably derived from dissections. Indeed the very meaning of the word anatomy is "to cut up the body." It is equally plausible to expect that the easily managed and accessible parts such as bones of the limbs should receive early and continuous study, and that the femur should be prominent among these.

Ward in 1838 and Wyman in 1857 were the first to advance the concept of the relationship between the orientation of the trabeculae of the cancellous bone and the external forces resisted by the bone. Culman and von Meyer reinforced this concept in 1867 by pointing out that the arrangement in the femur could be subject to mathematical analysis. Julius Wolff (1870) studied deformed bones and proclaimed that their trabecular arrangement reflected the same adaptation to the forces which deform them as the normal trabeculae bones responded to normal forces. The capacity to adapt to change was apparently inherent, at least in cancellous bone. Wolff formulated the law of bone formation which bears his name. This states that every "change in the form or function of a bone or of its function alone is followed by transformation of its internal architecture as well as changes in its external conformation in accordance with mathematical laws."

The above conclusions relating to transformation were derived principally from studies of ground scctions of boncs in which thc invcstigator could follow the course of trabeculae in the spongy parts (Fig. 25a). Whether similar conclusions may be valid regarding compact bones still is open to question, since the same method of study is not applicable.

However, in 1925 Benninghoff devised a technique that revealed the course of the Haversian systems in compact bone. He called it the "split line" method. Fresh bone was fixed in formalin and then decalcified in 5% nitric acid. After desiccation in

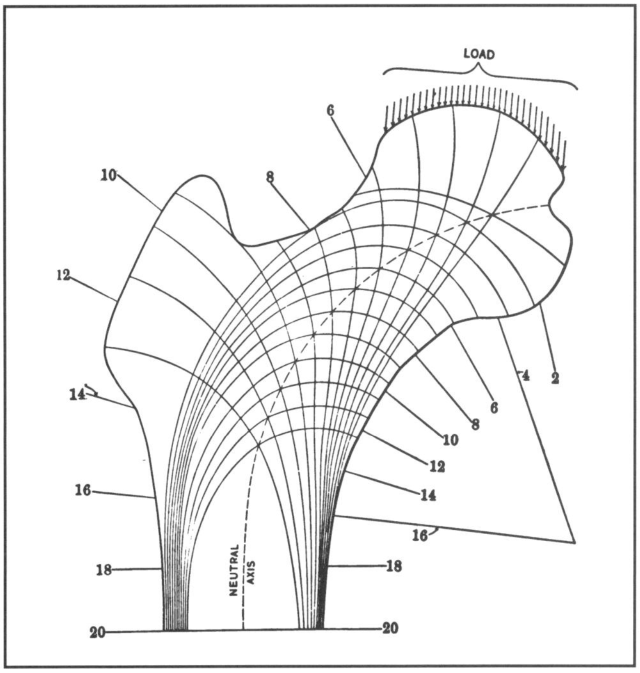

Fig. 25a. Diagram of lines of stress in the upper femur based on mathematical analysis (after Koch).

alcohol it was ready for study, but kept moist in 80% alcohol to prevent complete drying. The name "split line" derives from the method used in examining the specimen. This consisted of piercing the surface of the compact bone with a dull needle dipped in India ink in order to locate interlamellar lines, corresponding to the boundaries between Haversian systems. Having located such a line it was possible to create a crevice into which the ink would flow. By progressively separating the lamellae it was possible to lay out their courses in the compact bone. This yielded what has been interpreted as a diagram of force trajectories and when compared with those exhibited by the spicular arrangement of the spongiosa, the two appeared to be the same.

The analysis of the trajectories is not always as simple as might be assumed from the description of the technique; indeed the technique is of small value until the bone nears its mature stage and has attained a stable pattern. During its growing period it is undergoing widespread remodeling changes which exhibit a variety of transitory types of bone.

Only when this process slows down does Haversian system bone have time to form. Additional difficulties in interpretation of even mature bones are presented by the intricate patterns resulting from the variety of forces operating on a bone. These forces may differ in intensity, direction, and nature from either tension or compression. A further limitation is the fact that the split line technique can be applied only to *surfaces* of compact bones.

Analyses of the cranium have been made by a number of investigators beginning with Benninghoff, who laid out the general pattern of trajectories of the face and parts of the calvarium. Seipel wrote a comprehensive review of the literature on the subject and gave a detailed account of his own investigations of the trajectories of the jaws based on chimpanzee and human material. Havera (1961) studied the trajectories of the cranial base. This study was the subject of a thesis for the master of science degree and has never been published. It was a comparative anatomical study utilizing the horse, sheep, rabbit, cat, dog, monkey, and human. Since it bears on matters being discussed, some of the findings will be pointed out.

All animal life on the Earth exists in a gravitational field which exerts a continuous force on it. Only adaptations which provided means for resisting this force permitted animals to escape from a water environment and, stranded on land, to raise their bellies off the ground. Further adaptations permitted them to move, first on four legs, then on two legs and two arms (two legs and a tail), and eventually on two legs alone. Each of these demanded sweeping modifications of the skeleton, not only in the relative form, strength, and position of bones as a group, but within the individual bones as well. The most unremitting forces working on the skeleton are those involved in maintaining erect posture. These, therefore, are dominant in determining the trajectory of forces. Other systems such as those for movement and special functions are superimposed and may even tend to dominate in certain areas. The adaptations that have occurred in the cranial base with the change from the horizontal posture of four-footed animals to the upright posture of bipedal humans are numerous, but we need consider only a few.

The most obvious change is in the location of the foramen magnum. In four-footed animals, this large opening between the cranial cavity and the spinal canal faces almost directly posteriorly. It is flanked by the occipital condyles which form the bearing surfaces between the head and body and are located in the area of least movement. The leverage and resulting forces at the condyles are very great in an animal such as the horse, with its large long head. Heavy compression forces working in a forward direction are reflected in a massive pillar which has its base in the condyles and begins to divide only as it approaches the back of the face (Fig. 25b). The tensions which balance this force and prevent the head from dropping are provided by the ligaments and powerful dorsal muscles of the neck which cover the entire upper posterior surface of the head (Fig. 25c).

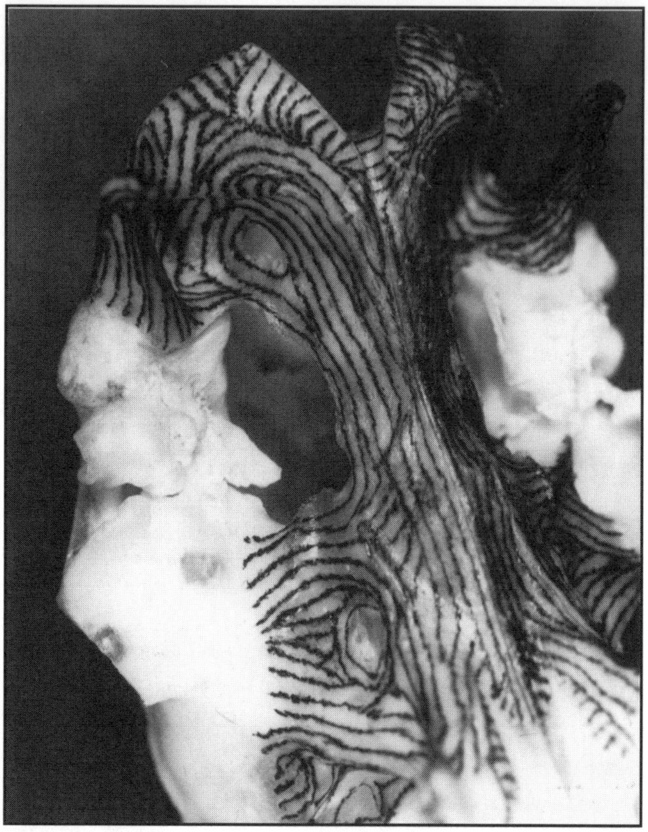

Fig. 25b. Split-line preparation of cranial base of horse showing strong midline pillar for transmission of occipital condylar forces (Havera).

The pattern in the sheep is similar to that of the horse, but not so strongly developed because the forces are less. The midline pillar still is a prominent characteristic (Fig. 25d), and the foramen is located somewhat lower and opens slightly more down-

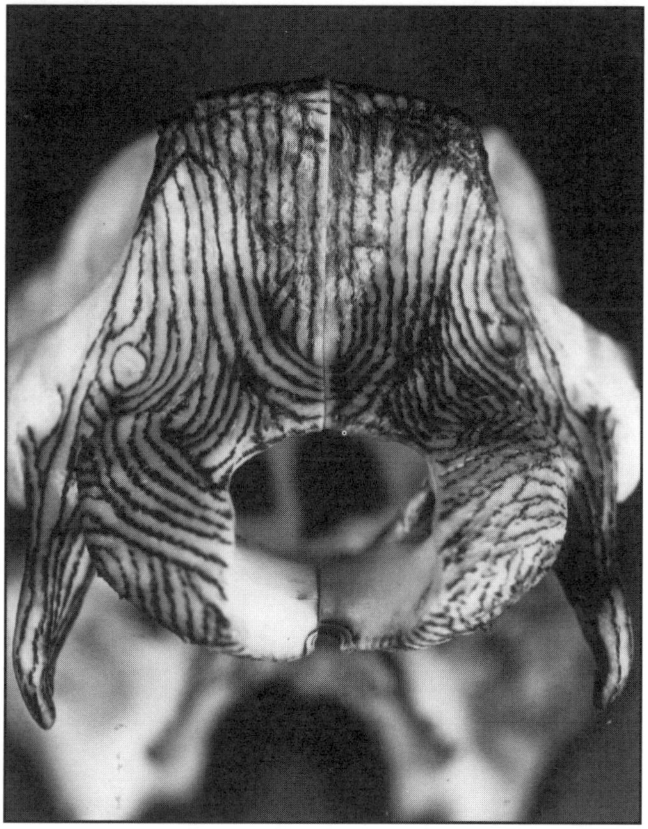

Fig. 25c. Split-line preparation of area around foramen magnum of horse reflecting muscle tension forces behind foramen (Havera).

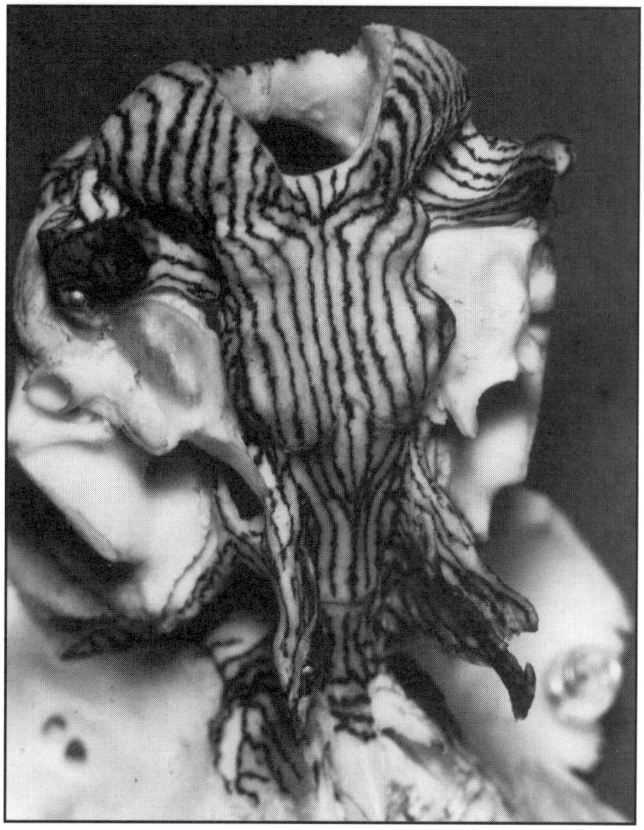

Fig. 25d. Split-line preparation of cranial base of sheep. Note similarity to pattern in horse (Havera).

ward (Fig. 25e). These differences may reflect the grazing posture which the sheep maintains for long periods of time.

Split-line preparation of the rabbit skull reflects differences associated with the more upright posture of this animal, which spends much time on its haunches. Both the foramen magnum and the condyles are located more downward and forward, lessening the compressive and tension forces. In keeping with these differences, the bone pattern is not so strongly marked even though the arrangement is the same (Fig. 25f).

The effects of the demands of the high degree of specialization necessary in those animals living on a carnivorous flesh diet can be seen in a wide range of adaptations. In the cats (Fig. 25g), the temporalis muscle has come to envelop most of the top and back of the head. It snaps the jaws together at great speed by operating on a coronoid process that extends high above the level of the zygomatic arch. In back, the temporalis attaches to the ridge which lies at the junction of the parietal and occipital bones. This same ridge also furnishes an anterior attachment for the dorsal muscles of the neck. The action of these muscles imposes heavy loads on the occipital condyles and sets up strong compression forces which can be visualized in split line preparations around foramen magnum (Fig. 25h) as well as in the anterior midline pillar.

Animals whose posture more nearly approaches the upright posture of humans, such as the monkeys and apes, show alterations that have long been taken to indicate the ascendancy of the brain over the other parts of the head. This does not infer any lessening in the demands for the essential needs for food and oxygen, but rather, alterations in the means for acquiring them. Simultaneously, we find the appearance of new functions such as speech, with all of these changes markedly influenced by the ever-present force of gravity.

Although some terrestrial animals had been able to climb trees by means of their claws and teeth, it remained for a small lemur to first exhibit the simple but revolutionary modification of the first digit

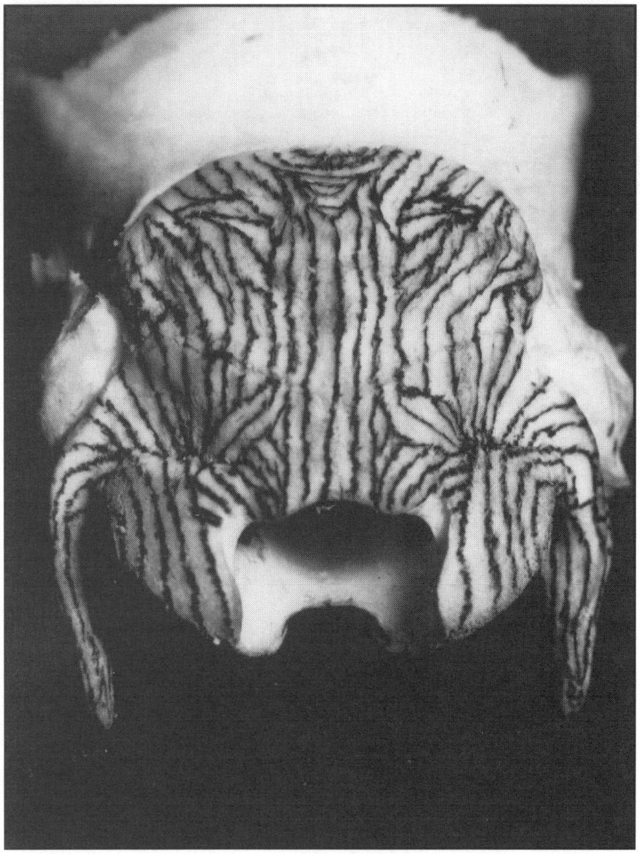

Fig. 25e. Split-line preparation of area behind foramen magnum in sheep (Havera).

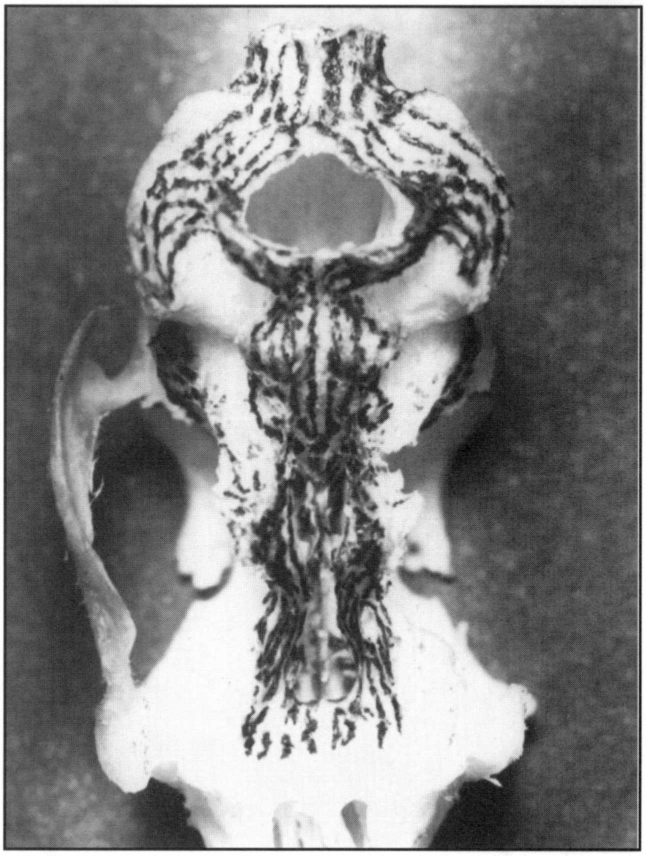

Fig. 25f. Split-line preparation of cranial base of rabbit. Relatively lighter pattern of midline pillar reflecting lighter compression forces (Havera).

of the forepaw that transformed the paw into a hand. This was the key that permitted grasping and the possibility of arboreal living. But the "opposable thumb" had more important implications for the animal than simple climbing and living in trees. It could now grasp objects and hold them before the face where the eyes, which had meanwhile moved from the side of the head to the front, could examine them with stereoscopic vision. All of these mutational changes added to demands on the brain and are held to be responsible for the subsequent selective increase in size of the brain.

As the forelimbs were relieved of more and more of their responsibility for locomotion, the hands assumed more of the function of food procurement as the jaws progressively retreated. These new feeding habits in turn required a new posture. The forward part of the body had to be maintained off the ground and held there during feeding without the help of the forelimbs. Partial adaptation to a more erect posture had already been attained through arboreal life, but conservation of energy demanded further modifications for a more complete terrestrial existence. This was particularly true in maintenance of the position of the head as it was undergoing great differential growth changes.

Weidenreich in his 1941 monograph "The Brain and Its Role In the Phylogenetic Transformation of the Human Skull," makes the point that the brain continues to increase in size with each stage of phylogenetic advance regardless of the type of changes occurring in other parts. Such increases are characterized by changes in its form as well as corresponding changes in the size and form of the skull that contains it. The brain becomes higher, wider, and longer and its general form more globular. The inner table of the skull follows these changes but the form of the outer table may depart markedly. For the most part, the external alterations reflect the demands of environmental forces of gravity and muscle tensions.

The significant increase in the size and weight of the brain was naturally accompanied by a change in its center of gravity, which gradually moved forward along with the foramen magnum and the occipital

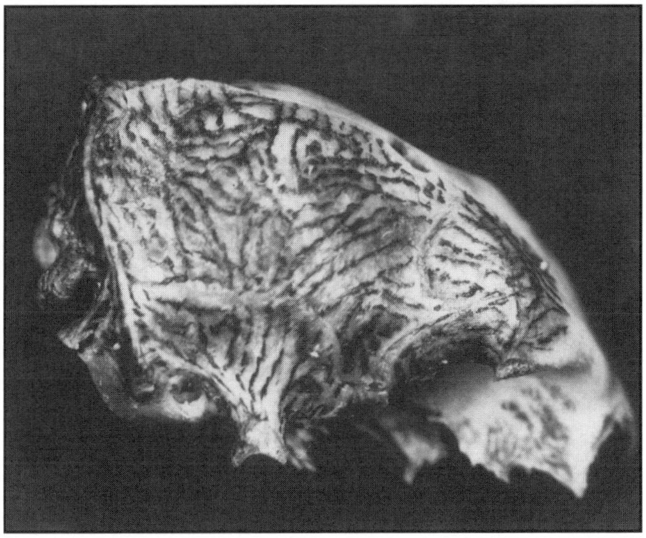

Fig. 25g. Split-line preparation of cat skull, lateral aspect. Note wide area of origin of temporalis muscle tension and the force-distribution (compression) arrangement supporting the glenoid fossa (Havera).

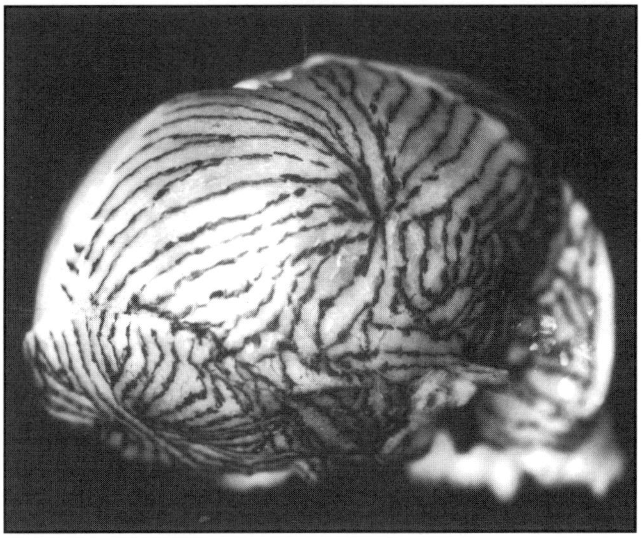

Fig. 25i. Split-line preparation of skull of macaque monkey to show striking change in shape with more upright posture (Havera).

condyles. The effects on these structures and upon those which assist them in resisting the forces acting upon them from different directions is reflected in the trajectoral systems of a split-line preparation of the macaque monkey (Fig. 25i). The most important new features are rounded contours of the skull

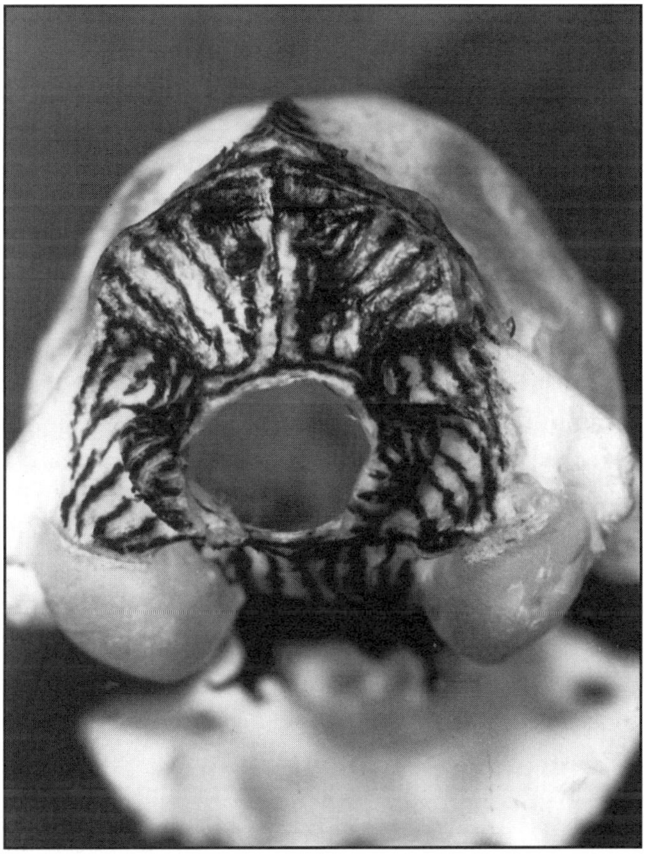

Fig. 25h. Split-line preparation of cat skull behind foramen magnum (Havera).

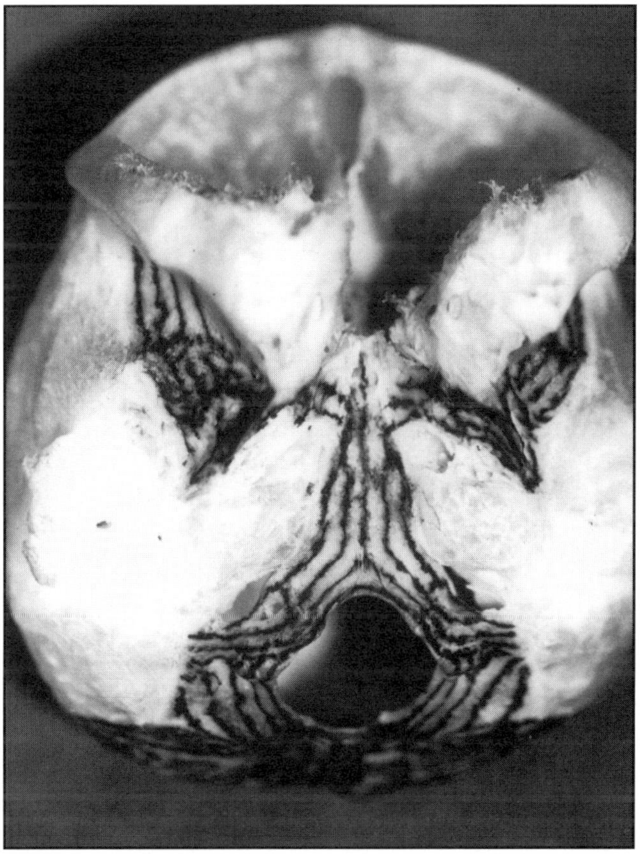

Fig. 25j. Split-line preparation of monkey skull showing lateral stress pathway over jugular process. (Havera)

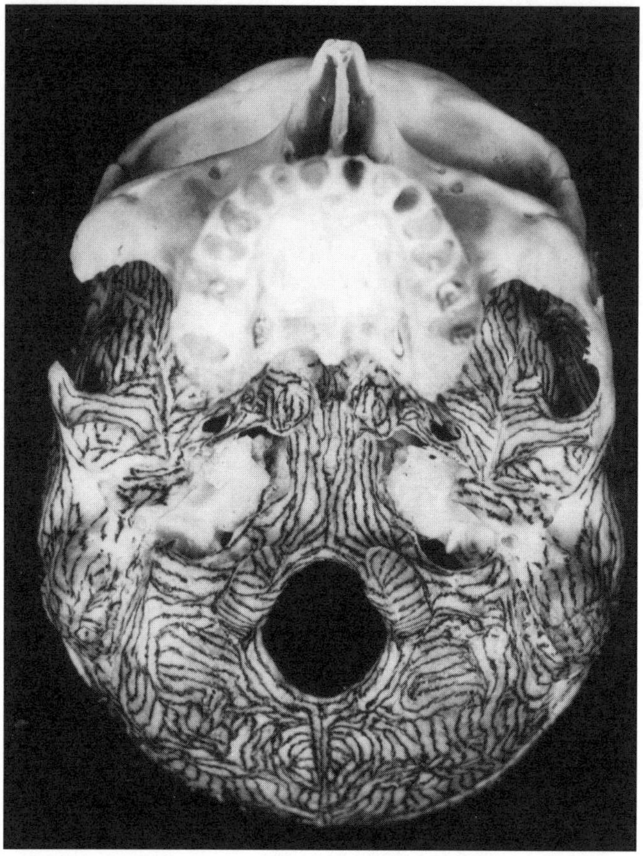

Fig. 25k. Split-line preparation of cranial base of human. Note that midline pillar passes its stresses bilaterally to the great wings of the sphenoid bone (Havera).

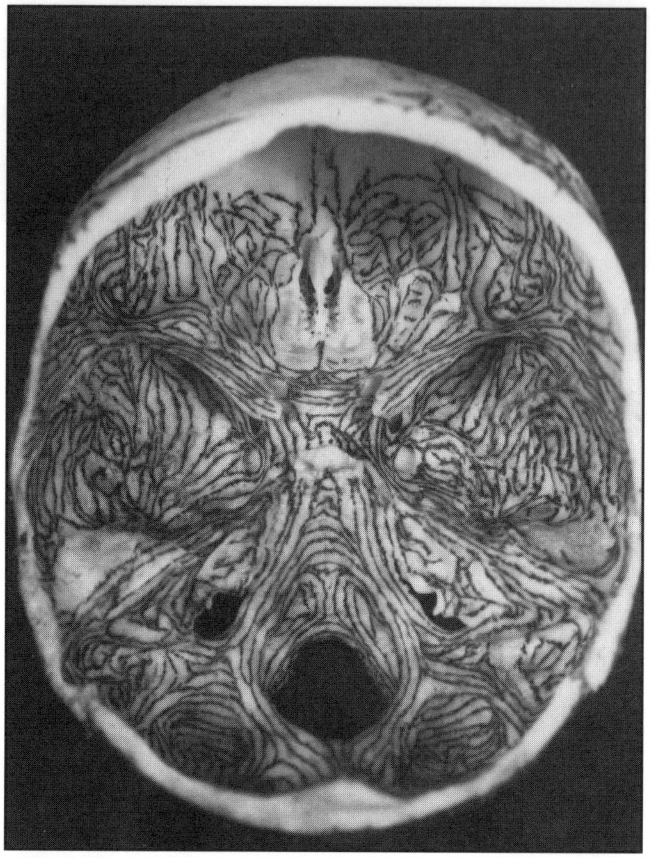

Fig. 25m. Split-line preparation of internal surface of human skull. Note courses of stress lines from foramen magnum (Havera).

and the more anterior position of foramen magnum. Posterior to this opening can be seen lines indicating trajectories coursing from the condyles upward across the occipital squama. Fig. 25k exhibits lines running laterally across the jugular process to the temporal bone. Forces carried forward through the body of the sphenoid bone are transferred to the great wings of that bone, thus protecting the delicate nasal septum and ethmoidal labyrinths which lie immediately forward of the sphenoid body.

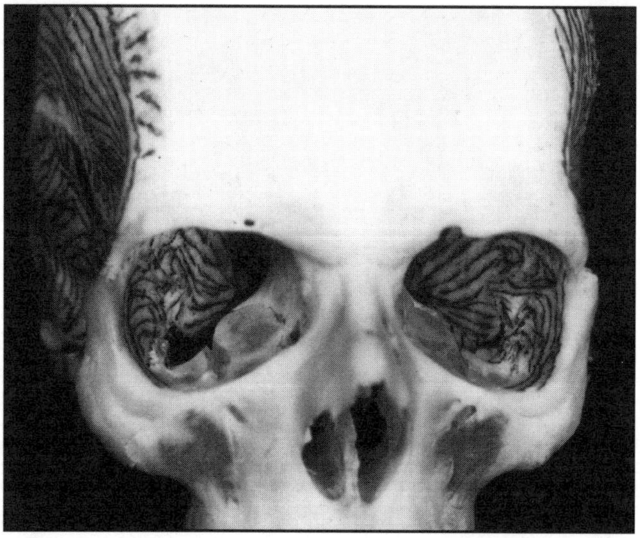

Fig. 25l. Split-line preparation of human stress line in the orbital surface of the great wing of the sphenoid bone (Havera)

A comparison of the basal view of the prepared human skull with the monkey skull shows the results of the attainment of fully erect posture. The human foramen magnum has moved still farther forward and downward and now opens in a slightly forward direction. The pattern of split lines around the foramen magnum behind the condyles is much the same as in the monkey, but the lines on the condylar surfaces reflect a more effective dispersal of forces laterally over the jugular buttress. Anteriorly, the condylar lines converge to pass forward through the basioccipital and sphenoid body. Again at the anterior limit of the sphenoid body the bearing of the stresses is assumed by the greater wings. Fig. 25k shows these lines as they continue into the lateral wall of the orbit, ending at right angles to the vertical trajectories of the frontal process of the zygomatic bone.

Split-line treatment of the internal surface of the cranial base shows a pattern uncomplicated by the evidence of those physical and functional forces revealed on the external surface. Only the structures and main division of the brain are reflected by the split lines (Fig. 25m).

Reading list:

Havera, James Ronald. *Stress line analysis of the base of the skull in animals and man by the split-line technique.* Thesis (MS in orthodontia), University of Illinois, 1961.

Koch, John C. "Laws of bone architecture." *American Journal of Anatomy,* 21:177, 1917.

26.

General Stress Pathways of the Head

It must be realized that there are two main systems through which stresses are conveyed around the head. One of these resists forces reaching the head from outside and the other resists forces arising within the head itself. Forces entering the head from outside do so principally from the occipital condyles or in jumping or from the calvarium in the case of blows.

Forces from the occipital condyle give rise to vectors in a radial manner which are transmitted over well-defined reinforced pathways due to the presence of foramina. The main course of these forces is directed forward and upward along the basilar part of the occipital bone and transmitted to the body of the sphenoid. Here, the greater wings of the sphenoid assume the stress and convey it toward the periphery in a forward, lateral, and upward direction to the outer table of the skull, where it is dissipated.

Forces falling on the head from above and in front are conveyed along these same pathways but in an opposite direction. However, a secondary pathway passes around the rim of the foramen magnum to the middle nuchal crest and the nuchal line to be ultimately dissipated over the outer table of the planum occipitale.

The forces that arise and are absorbed within the head are almost exclusively from mastication. These are not difficult to visualize. Forces from the maxillary incisor and canine teeth travel upward around the nasal aperture over the frontonasal process to dissipate on the outer table of the frontal bone. Those emanating from the premolar teeth and the first molar converge to pass up the maxillary and frontosphenoidal processes of the zygomatic bone, then move along the zygomatic process and toward the outer table of the frontal bone at the lateral boundary of the orbit. Here the "split-line" method of examining bone seems to indicate the forces divide, some travelling over the supraorbital margin but most arching upward and backward following the course of the temporal line.

More posterior forces from the molars or from the face itself follow the course of the zygomatic arch and ultimately reach the sturdy area where the squama of the temporal bone joins the posterior inferior angle of the parietal. From here, the stresses follow the temporal line as it arches upward and forward, forming a closed system of force distribution. Forces from teeth posterior to the first molars also are partially transmitted upward and backward and medially over the pterygoid process to the body of the sphenoid bone.

The study of dried skulls alone does not yield a complete picture of force distribution in the head. Although the "split-line" analysis reveals the course of Haversian systems and sheds light on the problem, there also is the complication of muscle stress which is resisted by bone. It is here that a limited application of electromyography is possible. Indeed, this technique strongly indicates that there are numerous situations in which the stresses on bone are resisted mainly by muscle, permitting the reduction of the bone to a minimum.

The Palatine Bone

Before leaving the upper face it is important that we consider the palatine bone, even though it is not an integral part of the force distribution system. Each palatine bone is "L" shaped when viewed from in front or back. The horizontal portion forms the posterior one-quarter of the hard palate, and its posterior edge in turn affords attachment for the palatine aponeurosis. The perpendicular portion lies against the nasal wall of the maxilla in back of the large opening of the maxillary sinus, which it helps to close. Two processes surmount the perpendicular plate, the orbital and sphenoidal. The orbital process is bent slightly laterally and its superior surface forms the most medial and posterior part of the orbital floor. The sphenoidal process follows the wall of the nose as it narrows superiorly and articulates with the inferior surface of the body of the sphenoid immediately in front of the medial pterygoid plate.

However, it is the pyramidal process which holds the greatest interest. This process arises from the perpendicular plate about the junction with the palatal or horizontal part. It follows the lower part of the posterior curvature of the maxilla to which it is connected by a suture. Posteriorly, the process presents a triangular concave surface, the lateral margins of which articulate with a like-shaped notch separating the pterygoid plates below. Sometimes the pyramidal process extends laterally far enough to be visible in the infratemporal fossa. At other times, the lateral pterygoid plate appears to meet the maxilla just above the tuberosity. The great importance of the pyramidal process lies in its vital relation to deglutition, a function which is even present before birth. Serial roentgenographic studies of children have shown that the pterygo-maxillary figure, formed by the back of the maxilla and the pterygoid process, remains stable after two and one-half to three years of age. The pyramidal process caught between these structures must also remain stable, thus maintaining stability of the soft palate.

The Mandible

The mandible is the largest and strongest single bone of the head. It is connected to the cranial skeleton only by ligaments and muscles. As with many bones, this bone has multiple functions—only one of which is mastication, perhaps the least vital in modern humans.

The fundamental framework of the mandible is a bone which curves downward and forward from its junction with the temporal bone to meet with its fellow from the opposite side of the symphysis. In many animals this is not a bony union, the two halves being joined by fibrous and elastic tissue. To this fundamental form, various processes have been added to give effectiveness to muscular action. For example, in the carnivore and similar animals of prey the coronoid process is highly developed. This structure provides attachment for the temporalis muscle which is oriented to provide rapid closure required by these animals. Indeed, the coronoid process may be found to extend well above the zygomatic arch.

The angular process likewise shows marked species differentiation. In the herbivorous and omnivorous animals, it tends to approach a right angle to serve the powerful masseter muscles. In the rodents, the angular process is greatly developed posteriorly to assist the specialized heads of the masseter muscles in protrusion of the jaw for incisal function.

A human is the only primate that has a chin, but *not* because a human is the only one to talk. Again, this adaptation is in the interest of muscular forces. As we shall see, on gaining an upright position, humans required marked modifications of the mandible to maintain that posture. For those of you interested in this fascinating story, it is suggested you read "The Adaptive Chin" (Du Brul & Sicher). The alveolar process is not a true part of the mandible in that it is derived from and dependent on the teeth for its existence. If no tooth germs form, as in anodontia, the alveolar process does not form and following the loss of teeth the same process tends to disappear. Neither do the teeth follow nor reflect the form of the lower border of the mandible. In the incisor region, where one might expect the bone to be thinner to match the teeth, the lower border of the mandible is thickest. These teeth and the alveolar process show wide variation in relationship to the lower border of the mandible, some being well forward and others well back, producing a pronounced mental eminence. Further back, where the broad surfaces and heavy loads of the molars would seem to require a heavy lower border, it is thinner than anywhere else. Here also the dental arch swings medial so that the last molar is completely medial to the ascending ramus.

The form of the mandible conforms to the internal stress placed upon it by muscular action. If the jaw is opened and protruded the action of the masseter muscles is to compress the ends of the "horse-shoe" shaped bone toward the midline. There is thus a resultant thickness reinforcement to prevent fracture at the midline of the mandible. As an illustration, a tightly fitted toothpick from the lingual of one mandibular molar to the same position on the opposite side of the dental arch will become increasingly tight if the mandible is opened and protruded.

Reading list:

Du Brul, E. Lloyd, and Sicher, Harry. *The Adaptive Chin.* Springfield, IL: Charles C. Thomas Publishers, 1954.

27.
The Dissipation of Dental Forces

Force trajectories of the face have received the attention of a number of investigators; Seipel has included a rather complete review and critique of their methods and findings in his monograph "Trajectories of the Jaws." Most of the early studies had been carried out by saving and grinding dried bones. But this approach showed only those structures lying in a single plane. Decalcification of bone followed by microdissection and the split-line application of dye permitted Seipel and later Havera to follow uneven surfaces as well as to determine the course of Haversian systems that ran in other than direct courses. For the present only the main trajectories of the outer bone surfaces of the face will be considered.

Since the outer surfaces of the maxilla are the main carriers of masticatory forces, it is interesting to note that although the course of most of the lines is perpendicular to the occlusal plane, they do not end at the necks of the teeth but rather in a zone that encircles that dental arch and exhibits a horizontal disposition of lines. Such an abrupt change of direction is subject to several possible interpretations.

I. The fact that the margins of the tooth sockets are alveolar rather than skeletal bones, and hence do not reveal a hereditary patterning.
II. The alveolar bone undergoes constant change throughout life in the interest of adjustment to tooth wear.
III. The stress borne by alveolar bone is one of tension while those working on the surfaces of the maxilla are of compression.

The lines running perpendicular to the alveolar zone follow courses which would be expected to resist forces emanating from the teeth. Those beginning above the anterior teeth course upward around the nasal notch and parallel the borders of the frontonasal process to the frontal bone. Lines above the first premolars tend to follow those from the incisors and canine, but those above the second premolar usually are weaker and less definitive. Lying under the canine fossa, an area designated as a neutral zone by Seipel, they tend to flow toward the anterior and posterior group or to disappear almost entirely. Their strength and direction may well be determined by facial type; i.e., long and narrow or short and wide. As yet, no studies have been made to determine whether such correlations exist.

As might be expected, the lines beginning above the first and second molars converge to pass upward and lateral-ward to follow the zygomatic process of the maxilla and the maxillary process of the zygomatic bone. Although the masticatory forces from the first molar must be transmitted upward to the frontal bone over the frontosphenoidal process of the zygomatic bone, the split-line technique does not reveal this to be the sole force operating. At the malar eminence, lines running from back, front, above, and below indicate the meeting of a number of forces in this area. Although most of these may be compressive there may be some due to muscle tensions, since this bone also provides attachment for the powerful masseter.

At the back of the dental arch, the lines tend to travel more posteriorly so that they may be seen on the lateral surface of the pyramidal process of the palatine bone and even more strongly on the medial surface. These later diverge slightly as they travel across the palatine shelves to meet those of the other side. A similar transpalatal series of lines can be found in the anterior part of the palate. Barth reported transverse trajectories throughout the palate on the basis of x-ray pictures.

A moment's reflection on what has been discussed above leads one to the conclusion that only the outer surface of the bones of the upper face can be considered skeletal in function. The maxilla, which constitutes the greatest part, can support only the weakest of forces except at three major attachment points. These are near the midline at the function of the outer table of the frontal bone and on both sides at the back medially with the pterygoid process and laterally with the zygomatic arch. It is completely free at all other points of its periphery except for the paper-thin junction of its orbital surface with the lamina papybracea of the ethmoid labyrinth. Its skeletal role is largely one of protection, support, and separation of soft tissues. Although incapable of movement from the muscles attached to it, the maxilla transmits some of the heaviest functional forces of the body—those of mastication. Just like the dissipation of forces in the cranial base, those arising from the teeth are carried over sturdy buttresses to cranial areas of resistance, skirting the vital contents of the nasal and orbital cavities.

The mandible is a bone of a different sort. Although complementary to the maxilla in its masticatory function, it definitely belongs to the supportive skeleton in other respects. In humans, it plays a major role in postural maintenance, and its position in space is largely determined by muscles. The mandible has been studied more intensively than any other bone with the possible exception of the femur, perhaps due to its independence and accessibility. In spite of this, it still remains an enigma.

At birth, the mandible resembles a curved, tubular bone consisting of two halves. The connective tissue joining the two halves at the midline is replaced by bone during the first year of life. It is thought that this curved tubular bone extending from the symphysis to the temporomandibular joint provides the basal trajectoral system for the mandible. Superimposed on this basic structure are the secondary trajectoral systems of the coronoid, the angular processes, and the chin. These show marked variations in development among the species and reflect differences in prehensile and masticatory habits of the associated musculature.

Since action and reaction are equal and opposite, the mandible must withstand the same forces as the maxilla. It does this in a different manner, however. While the maxilla transmits its forces over buttresses that protect delicate parts, the mandible absorbs its forces and transfers them directly to its suspensory muscles. There are other forces of a different nature than the intermittent shocks of mastication which the mandible shares with the maxilla. The mandible is an important base of attachment for the antagonists of the antigravitational muscles of the postcervical region and is subject to the continuous pull of those muscles running to it from above and below. Even in the newborn, the basic trajectoral pattern is discernible in split-line preparations, foretelling those that characterize the adult. The mandibles of animals show striking adaptive changes accompanying the change in body posture. Limiting our attention to the lower border, we see in lower animals in outline proportionately smaller and narrower than in man. Both the inner and outer surfaces of the lower border show equally important changes, with the inner surface probably reflecting the more critical demands of respiration and deglutition.

At this point, the reader should attempt to imagine the results of an abrupt change of a four-footed animal to an upright posture. Even granting that the foramen magnum and occipital condyles have moved forward so that there would be no neural interference at the junction of the head and the body, there would be disastrous consequences anteriorly involving breathing and swallowing. The forward thrust of the column of the neck between the rami of the mandible would jam the hyoid bone and the tongue forward, closing both air and food channels.

Du Brul and Sicher, in their monograph "The Adaptive Chin," have nicely demonstrated progressive changes in the mandible that mark the transformation from monkeys to humans. These show a gradual increase in proportional size from a stage at which the dentition can be seen to lie completely outside of the mandible perimeter to man where it lies completely inside. This relative widening and shortening of the mandible is accompanied by changes in the musculature of the region related to changes in the position of the hyoid bone as it moves forward with the column of the neck. The tongue becomes gradually more rounded, particularly from front to back as the mouth cavity is reshaped accordingly. The anterior bellies of the digastric muscle offer the chief aid to gravity in opening the mouth in monkeys. They diverge from their midline attachment to the hyoid at an acute angle to each other as they run forward to attach on the lower border of the mandible close to the midline. As the mandible widens, these muscles tend to become more parallel and to attach even more laterally on the hyoid bone until in humans the tendons connecting their anterior and posterior bellies are completely lateral to the hyoid bone and connected to it by only a fascial loop.

To this author, the muscles which seem to have adapted most effectively to the eversion of the lower border of the mandible are the geniohyoids.

This pair of muscles is attached close to the midline on the inner surface of the mandible immediately above the mylohyoid—the muscular floor of the mouth. In increasing in thickness as they proceed backward and slightly downward, they claim almost the entire anterior surface of the hyoid bone for their insertion. These muscles play the chief part in holding the hyoid bone, larynx, and tongue forward and free of the vertebral column when the animal is in the upright posture, thus maintaining the anteroposterior dimension of the airway. More will be said about these muscles in appropriate sections. It is sufficient here to realize that the human, the only vertically oriented mammal, is also the only one having a chin and that this chin is his most ventrally located skeletal point.

Reading list:

Benninghoff, A. "Splatlinien am Knocken, leine Methodezur Ermottlung der Architektur platter Knochen." *Verb. Anat. Ges.*, 1925.

Enlow, D.H. *Principles of Bone Remodelling*. Springfield, IL: Charles C. Thomas Publishers, 1963.

Gregory, W.K. "Williston's Law, relating to the evolution of skull bones in the vertebrates." *American Journal of Physical Anthropology*, 20, July-Sept. 1938.

Koch, J.C. "The laws of bone architecture." *American Journal of Anatomy,* 21: 127-129, 1917.

Seipel, G. *Trajectories of the Jaws.* P.A. Norstedt & Soner, 1948.

Ward, F.O. *Outlines of Human Osteology*. London: Henry Renshaw, 1836.

Weinman, J.P. & Sicher, H. *Bone and Bones.* 2nd ed. St. Louis, MO: C.V. Mosby Co., 1955.

Wolff, J. "Uber die innere Architectur der Knocken und ihre Bedeutung fur die Frage von Knochenewachstum." *Virchows Arch.,* 50: 389-450, 1870.

________. "Das Gesetz der Transformation der Knochen." Berlin, 1892.

Wyman, J. "On the cancellous structure of some of the bones of the human body." *Boston Journal of Natural History,* 6: 125-140, 1857.

"Evolution of dental occlusion from fish to man." University of Pennsylvania Bicentennial Conference, 1941.

28. Orthodontia and Root Resorption

Orthodontic tooth movement and root resorption came to be associated in orthodontic thinking largely as the result of Ketcham's report in 1923. One factor after another was advanced, all based on the assumption that appliances were the prime contributors to the etiology of root resorption. "Jiggling" of the teeth, excessive force, rigidity of arch attachment by bracket, rapid treatment, and prolonged treatment all were suggested as causes before nonmechanical factors were considered.

Oppenheim (1935 and 1936) demonstrated that the x-ray was not a completely reliable method for the detection of resorption except at the apex, and also that the light forces exercised by finger springs were as likely to be associated with resorption as were other, heavier forces. He proved these points in the following manner:

Teeth which had been marked for extraction were first moved lingually or buccally with either arch and ligatures or with lingual arches. Following extraction, they were decalcified and completely sectioned in series. They were then reconstructed according to the technique of Born, which provides a greatly enlarged model perfectly proportioned in three planes of space. The figures illustrate the striking evidence of resorption, none of which would be discernible from an intraoral film.

With the support of a grant from the American Association of Orthodontists, Marshall conducted tooth-moving experiments on monkeys. In spite of forces greatly in excess of those used in orthodontics, he could not demonstrate root resorption in the animals on normal diets. It was evident, however, in monkeys on diets deficient in certain essentials. Examining patients in a hospital devoted to endocrine disorders, Becks found a high incidence of root resorption in comparison to that of other hospital populations.

Cases from private practices were reported in which there had been no orthodontic treatment and indeed, there were those in which marked generalized attenuation of the roots had been unsuspected until revealed by x-rays late in life. On the other hand were those cases in which all precautions had been ignored, e.g., "jiggling," heavy forces, fast or greatly prolonged treatment, all without development of discernible damage. These cases have been classified as ideopathic, but the question might be raised whether or not this term might not be applied to all cases of root resorption with equal justification. It seems evident that constitutional factors alone can be responsible in some cases, and may be contributory to all in which resorption occurs.

In the face of such a large mass of diverse evidence, the orthodontist has few guides for his mechanical treatment. However, a review of the work of investigators and clinicians alike reveals consensus if not proof on the following points:

I. No force that causes pain should be applied.

II. Treatment should be started with the lightest force possible.

III. This force should be allowed to operate for sufficient time to permit the initial slackening of the periodontal ligament fibers and the appearance of osteoclasts (a minimum of one week).

IV. A lack of expected movement does not indicate the need for increased force; on the contrary, it calls for more time for the force to operate.

V. Recovery periods should be allowed following periods of movement. This is particularly true of elastic forces.

VI. That portion of the periodontal ligament lying nearest to the alveolar crest is the main retention apparatus of the tooth. Teeth that have suffered the loss of the apical one-half or even more of their roots remain firm, while those that lose attachment near the surface quickly become loose.

VII. Although it is generally accepted that the fibers of the ligament are nonextensible themselves, the fact that their terminals overlap and lie next to each other in the ground substance permits stretching of the ligament by an alteration of the chemical bonds which hold them together at rest. A tooth may be moved appreciably if pressure is maintained upon it steadily for but a few minutes, provided the pressure remains below the pain threshold. Force above this level results in a tearing of the ligament.

29.

Gubernaculum: The Second Dentition

As early as the eighteenth century, John Hunter called attention to small openings lying lingual to the deciduous teeth in young humans. Hunter wrote, "when the incisors are little advanced but long before they appear through their bony sockets there are small holes leading to them on the inside or behind the temporary sockets and teeth, and these holes grow larger and larger till at last the body of the tooth passes quite through them." The little holes were given the name "gubernaculum" openings and their contents gubernacular cords. As Scott has pointed out, their discovery was the result of dissections by anatomists.

With the advent of the microscope and the accompanying preparation of thin tissue sections, these small structures were lost sight of and their importance unrecognized. Attention has since been focused on them by Brash, and Scott has employed combined dissection and histologic techniques for their study. The most recent report is that of Carrollo, Hoffman, and Brodie who used a similar combination of methods.

Dissection of the lingual side of the mandible of young pigs with complete primary dentition revealed the secondary lamina lying at the level of or just below the alveolar crest in the region of the buccal teeth. Manipulation revealed it to be a tough, fibrous band attached to the periosteum of the jaw. This was obviously a gubernacular cord. Anterior to the first deciduous molar it travelled forward across the diastema on the superior surface of the mandible to the canine where it entered the lingual plate of the mandible. Previous studies had shown that there were no gubernacular openings in the bone surface lingual to the lower primary incisors in the pig. However, extraction of those teeth from dried skulls of the same age revealed them in the lingual wall of the tooth sockets.

Opposite the bifurcation of the roots of each of the buccal teeth there was a hole in the lingual wall just below its free margin. This gubernacular opening ran down to the follicle of the permanent tooth.

Fig. 29a is a buccolingual section of the mandible in the region of the bifurcation of the premolar roots, alongside a labelled drawing. It reveals one-half of the primary tooth still retained in the alveolar bone. Beneath this can be seen alveolar bone in the middle of which is the gubernacular canal. Note that this opens on the lingual side of the alveolar process above. At the bottom of the canal can be seen the bud of the permanent tooth, which is beginning to calcify. It is surmounted by a cone-like epithelial structure which makes a direct connection with the outer enamel epithelium of the germ. Above its apex it joins with a cord coming down through the gubernacular canal. In Fig. 29b. is seen a horizontal microscopic section of the canal and its contents, the most striking aspect of which is

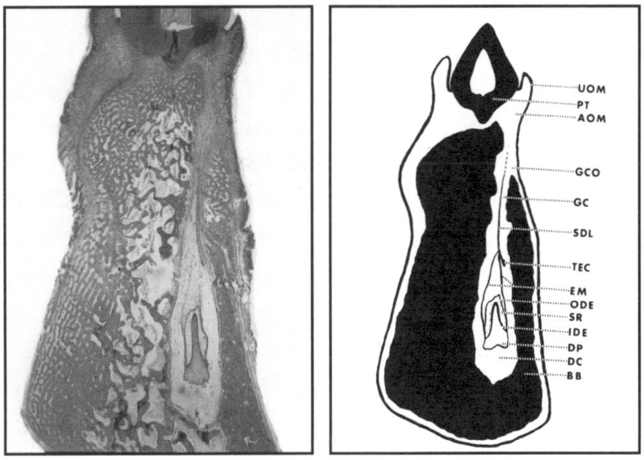

Fig. 29a.

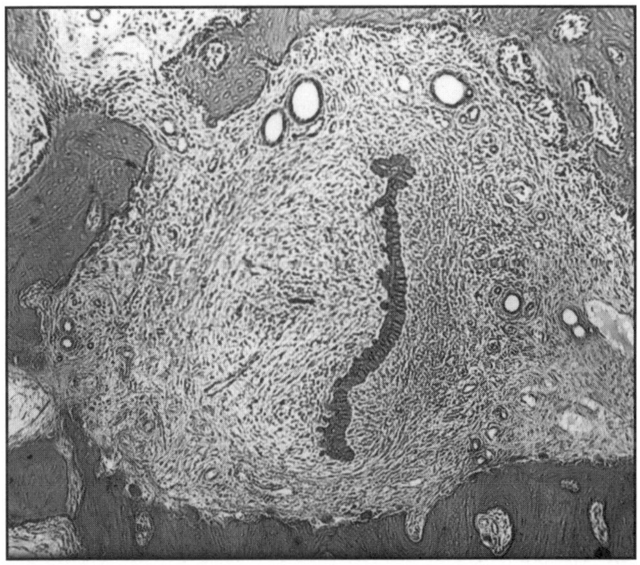

Fig. 29b.

the centrally located accumulation of cells. These are epithelial cells arranged two or three cells deep and 60-70 cells wide.

A frontal section shows them running from the submucosa of the mouth above the bony canal opening down the gubernacular canal to a cluster of cells just above the germ of the second tooth. Immediately adjacent to this nodule is the cone of epithelium connected to the outer enamel epithelium. It is but one cell thick as it descends to join with the epithelium of the tooth crown around its periphery. Cells within the cone resemble those of the stellate reticulum, except that they are more densely packed.

Connective tissue surrounds the epithelium of the gubernacular cord, organized into an inner and outer layer. The inner layer approximates the epithelium while the outer layer intervenes between the inner wall and the bony wall of the gubernacular canal. The collagen fibers of the inner layer are oriented parallel to the long axis of the epithelium. They are of greater density on the medial aspect of the chord than they are on the lateral. Only small capillaries are found on the inner layer.

In the outer layer the density of the collagen fibers is less and the collagen fiber orientation is more random. Many osteoclasts are seen on the bony border throughout the length of the posterolateral aspect of the gubernacular canal. Conversely, many osteoclasts are observed along the entire anteromedial aspects of the bony canal. Many larger arteries and veins run parallel to the long axis of the canal in the outer layer of connective tissue. The connective tissues which surround the epithelium of the cord form a continuous connection between the connective tissue of the oral mucosa and that of the dental sac which surrounds the developing tooth.

As in so many embryological phenomenon it is impossible to state with certainty which tissues induce certain reactions in others in the development of the gubernacular system. Epithelium seems to be primary because each of its changes in age, form, and location witnesses specific changes in the potentials of the undifferentiated mesenchyme with which it is in contact. Its proliferation along a free border of the jaws to form the dental lamina and the tooth buds is accompanied in specific localities by histodifferential and morphodifferential changes in the mesenchyme which in turn are followed by the formation of dentin. This is thought to be due to the activity of the cells of the inner enamel epithelium.

The cells of the outer enamel epithelium and those forming the epithelial core of the gubernacular extensions connecting the enamel organ with the mucosa of the mouth are associated with changes in their surrounding mesenchyme that lead to quite different ends. This is the tissue which connects the submucosal connective tissue of the mouth with that of the dental sac encapsulating the tooth germ.

It might be compared to insulation surrounding the total epithelial components but it displays potentials far beyond those of passive insulation. It appears to establish and maintain the size of the gubernacular canal against the encroachment of the growing alveolar bone around it. This is shown by the experimental extirpation of the soft tissue from the canal which is quickly followed by the invasion of new alveolar bone resulting in loss of the connection between tooth germ and mouth.

Another aspect of its activity relates to the positional adjustment of the canal and tooth follicles to the growth of the jaws. It has been shown that the growth of the mandible and maxilla is in a general backward and outward direction, i.e., with periosteal bone added to the posterior and lateral surfaces. Such growth, expressed against relatively fixed cranial areas, is an important contributor to the forward and outward development of the facial skeleton. It might be expected that all structures contained within the maxilla and mandible would move with them. Microscopic studies reveal that this is true at least to the extent that original proportions are maintained.

The general pattern of the growth of the jaw bones is covered elsewhere in this book; consideration will be given here only to the contribution of the alveolar processes to their maturation.

As was shown in the previous sections, a trough of bone is built around developing tooth germs to a height beyond that of their occlusal surfaces. The edges of the trough do not close over the teeth because of the presence of the dental lamina. When the lamina is not present, as is presumably the case in ectodermal dysplasia with congenital absence of the teeth, the edges meet and the mandibular body forms a hollow shaft similar to that of a long bone.

The crowns of the primary teeth are normally partly calcified at birth and lie in the trough already separated from each other by thin partitions of bone.

The development and positioning of the upper teeth is essentially the same as in the lower. The second deciduous molar lies at or even above the level of the palate. The first permanent molar as seen in some x-rays is located behind and above, deeper than the roots of the second primary molar and just anterior to the pterygomaxillary fissure.

Appendix I.

Illustration Credits

A good faith effort has been made to find and credit the sources of the illustrations used in *The Dentofacial Complex*. With the passage of time since Dr. Allan G. Brodie used these illustrations in his lectures, however, some sources were impossible to find. We regret any errors or omissions.

Because many of these materials were created 40 or more years ago and were gathered from secondary sources and archives, it was not always possible to locate the copyright owners and secure their permission for use in this book. Permissions have been obtained to the extent possible. Should the reader recognize the work of an author, photographer, or graphic artist not listed in the text or bibliography, we would gratefully appreciate having it brought to our attention.

Foreword

Fig. Foreword-a: Collection of University of Illinois at Chicago College of Dentistry.

Fig. Foreword-b: Collection of University of Illinois at Chicago College of Dentistry Department of Orthodontics.

Preface

Collection of Dr. Abe Goldstein.

Fig. Preface-a: Gray, Henry; and Clemente, Carmine D (editor). *Anatomy of the Human Body,* 30th Edition. Philadelphia: Lea & Febiger, 1985. With permission from Lippincott Williams & Wilkins, Philadelphia, PA.

Chapter 2

Fig. 2a: Gregory, William King. *Evolution Emerging, Vol. II.* New York: Macmillan Co., 1951. Drawing by Helen Ziska. American Museum of Natural History Library.

Chapter 3

Fig. 3a: Negus, Victor E. *The Comparative Anatomy and Physiology of the Larynx.* London: Wm. Heinemann Medical Books Ltd., 1949.

Fig. 3b: Negus, Victor E. *The Comparative Anatomy and Physiology of the Larynx.* London: Heinemann Medical Books Ltd., 1949.

Fig. 3c: Negus, V.E. *The Comparative Anatomy and Physiology of the Larynx.* London: Heinemann Medical Books Ltd., 1949.

Fig. 3d: Collection of University of Illinois at Chicago College of Dentistry Department of Orthodontics.

Fig. 3e: Durzo, Carmine. *Growth behavior of the hyoid bone: a serial x-ray study.* Thesis (MS in orthdontia), University of Illinois, 1961.

Fig. 3f: Durzo, Carmine. *Growth behavior of the hyoid bone: a serial x-ray study*. Thesis (MS in orthdontia), University of Illinois, 1961.

Fig. 3g: Durzo, Carmine. *Growth behavior of the hyoid bone: a serial x-ray study.* Thesis (MS in orthdontia), University of Illinois, 1961.

Fig. 3h: Collection of University of Illinois at Chicago College of Dentistry Department of Orthodontics.

Chapter 4

Fig. 4a: Subtelny, Jacob Daniel. *Width of the Nasopharynx and Related Anatomical Structures in Normal and Unoperated Cleft Palate Children.* Thesis (MS in orthodontia), University of Illinois, 1953.

Fig. 4b: Kincaid, Robert Myron. *The frequency of deglutition in man; its relationship to overbite*. Thesis (MS in orthodontia), University of Illinois, 1949.

Chapter 5

Fig. 5a: Collection of University of Illinois at Chicago College of Dentistry Department of Orthodontics.

Fig. 5b: Gray, Henry; and Clemente, Carmine D (editor). *Anatomy of the Human Body,* 30th Edition. Philadelphia: Lea & Febiger, 1985. With permission from Lippincott Williams & Wilkins, Philadelphia, PA.

Chapter 6

Fig. 6a: Brodie, Allan G. Seminar notes, Oct. 26, 1949.

Fig. 6b: Gregory, William King. *Evolution Emerging, Vol. II*. New York: Macmillan Co., 1951. Drawing by Helen Ziska. American Museum of Natural History Library.

Fig. 6c: Drawing by Helen Ziska. American Museum of Natural History Library.

Fig. 6d: Collection of Dr. Allan G. Brodie.

Fig. 6e: Collection of University of Illinois at Chicago College of Dentistry Department of Orthodontics.

Fig. 6f: Collection of University of Illinois at Chicago College of Dentistry Department of Orthodontics.

Chapter 7

Fig. 7a: Collection of Dr. Allan G. Brodie.

Fig. 7b: Collection of Dr. Allan G. Brodie.

Fig. 7c: Collection of Dr. Allan G. Brodie.

Fig. 7d: Collection of Dr. Allan G. Brodie.

Fig. 7e: Collection of Dr. Allan G. Brodie.

Fig. 7f: Collection of Dr. Allan G. Brodie.

Fig. 7g: Collection of Dr. Allan G. Brodie.

Fig. 7h: Collection of Dr. Allan G. Brodie.

Chapter 8

Fig. 8a: Carlson, Harry. *Studies on the rate and amount of eruption of certain human teeth.* Thesis (MS in orthodontia), University of Illinois, 1942.

Fig. 8b: Collection of University of Illinois at Chicago College of Dentistry.

Fig. 8c: Collection of Dr. Allan G. Brodie.

Fig. 8d: Collection of Dr. Allan G. Brodie.

Fig. 8e: Collection of University of Illinois at Chicago College of Dentistry Department of Orthodontics.

Fig. 8f: Broadbent, B.H. "Ontogenetic Development of Occlusion." *Angle Orthodontist,* 11: 223-241, 1941. Courtesy the E.H. Angle Education and Research Foundation.

Fig. 8g: Collection of Dr. Allan G. Brodie.

Fig. 8h: Collection of University of Illinois at Chicago College of Dentistry Department of Orthodontics.

Fig. 8i: Collection of University of Illinois at Chicago College of Dentistry Department of Orthodontics.

Fig. 8j: Collection of University of Illinois at Chicago College of Dentistry Department of Oral and Maxillofacial Surgery.

Fig. 8k: Ortiz Paiz, Manuel Higinio. *On the growth of the human head from birth to the third month of life.* Thesis (MS in orthodontia), University of Illinois, 1945.

Fig. 8l: Dempster, W.T., Adams, W.J., Duddles, R.A. "Arrangement in the jaws of the roots of the teeth." *Journal of the American Dental Association.* 67(6):779-97, 1963. Figures 9 and 10. Copyright © 1963 American Dental Association. All rights reserved/Adapted 2004 with permission of the American Dental Association.

Fig. 8m: Mason, Jack. *Behavior of the axes of human molar teeth during growth and eruption.* Thesis (MS in orthodontia), University of Illinois, 1962.

Chapter 9

Fig. 9a: Steadman, S., and Schour, I. "Geometric construction of the rat incisor," *Journal of Dental Research,* 15:222 1935. Reprinted with permission from the *Journal of Dental Research.*

Chapter 11

Fig. 11a: Collection of Dr. Allan G. Brodie.

Fig. 11b: *Manual of Telephone Extension Program*, "Current Advances in Dentistry." Chicago: University of Illinois, 1949.

Fig. 11c: Collection of University of Illinois at Chicago College of Dentistry Department of Orthodontics.

Fig. 11d: Du Brul, E. Lloyd, and Sicher, Harry. *The Adaptive Chin.* Springfield, IL: Charles C. Thomas Publishers, 1954.

Chapter 13

Fig. 13a: Durzo, Carmine. *Growth behavior of the*

hyoid bone: a serial x-ray study. Thesis (MS in orthdontia), University of Illinois, 1961.

Fig. 13b: Collection of University of Illinois at Chicago Department of Orthodontics.

Fig. 13c: Collection of University of Illinois at Chicago College of Dentistry Department of Orthodontics.

Chapter 14
All photos courtesy of Dr. Lawrence Furstman.

Chapter 15
Fig. 15a: Collection of University of Illinois at Chicago College of Dentistry Department of Orthodontics.

Fig. 15b: Collection of University of Illinois at Chicago College of Dentistry Department of Orthodontics.

Fig. 15c: Collection of University of Illinois at Chicago College of Dentistry Department of Orthodontics.

Fig. 15d: Collection of University of Illinois at Chicago College of Dentistry Department of Orthodontics.

Fig. 15e: Collection of Dr. Allan G. Brodie.

Fig. 15f: Drawing by Dr. Massis A. Bahador, collection of University of Illinois at Chicago College of Dentistry Department of Orthodontics.

Chapter 17
Fig. 17a: Collection of University of Illinois at Chicago College of Dentistry Department of Orthodontics.

Fig. 17b: Reprinted from Brodie, Allan G., "Cephalometric Roentgenology: History, Technics, and Uses." *Journal of Oral Surgery*, 7: 185-198, 1949, with permission from the American Association of Oral and Maxillofacial Surgeons.

Fig. 17c: Collection of University of Illinois at Chicago College of Dentistry Department of Orthodontics.

Fig. 17d: Brodie, Allan G. "On the Growth Pattern of the Human Head from the Third Month to the Eighth Year of Life." *American Journal of Anatomy*, 68: 209-262, ©1941, Wiley. Reprinted by permission of Wiley-Liss, Inc., a subsidiary of Wiley & Sons Inc.

Fig. 17e: Reprinted from Brodie, Allan G., "Cephalometric Roentgenology: History, Technics, and Uses." *Journal of Oral Surgery,* 7: 185-198, 1949, with permission from the American Association of Oral and Maxillofacial Surgeons.

Fig. 17f: Collection of University of Illinois at Chicago College of Dentistry Department of Orthodontics.

Fig. 17g: Brodie, Allan G. "On the Growth Pattern of the Human Head from the Third Month to the Eighth Year of Life." *American Journal of Anatomy,* 68: 209-262, © 1941, Wiley. Reprinted by permission of Wiley-Liss, Inc., a subsidiary of Wiley & Sons Inc.

Fig. 17h: Reprinted from Brodie, Allan G., "Cephalometric Roentgenology: History, Technics, and Uses." *Journal of Oral Surgery*, 7: 185-198, 1949, with permission from the American Association of Oral and Maxillofacial Surgeons.

Fig. 17i: Collection of University of Illinois at Chicago College of Dentistry Department of Orthodontics.

Chapter 18
Fig. 18a: Hamilton, W.J., Boyd, J.D., Mossman, H.W. *Human Embryology.* Baltimore: The Williams & Wilkins Co., 1952. With permission from Lippincott Willliams & Wilkins, Philadelphia, PA.

Chapter 21
Fig. 21a: Gregory, William King. *Our Face from Fish to Man.* New York: Hafner Publishing Co., Inc., 1963.

Chapter 22
Fig. 22a: Moore, Alton. *Head growth of the Macaque monkey as revealed by vital staining, embedding, and undecalcified sections.* Thesis (MS in orthodontia), University of Illinois, 1948.

Fig. 22b: Scheiman-Tagger, Etty, and Brodie, Allan G. "Lead Acetate as a Marker of Growing Calcified Tissues. A Modified Method." *Anatomical Record,* 150(4): 439, 1964. Press of the Wistar Institute of Anatomy and Biology, Philadelphia, PA.

Chapter 23

Fig. 23a: Gray, Henry; and Clemente, Carmine D (editor). *Anatomy of the Human Body,* 30th Edition. Philadelphia: Lea & Febiger, 1985. With permission from Lippincott Williams & Wilkins, Philadelphia, PA.

Fig. 23b: Gray, Henry; and Clemente, Carmine D (editor). *Anatomy of the Human Body,* 30th Edition. Philadelphia: Lea & Febiger, 1985. With permission from Lippincott Williams & Wilkins, Philadelphia, PA.

Fig. 23c: Gray, Henry; and Clemente, Carmine D (editor). *Anatomy of the Human Body,* 30th Edition. Philadelphia: Lea & Febiger, 1985. With permission from Lippincott Williams & Wilkins, Philadelphia, PA.

Fig 23d: Gray, Henry; and Clemente, Carmine D (editor). Anatomy of the Human Body, 30th Edition. Philadelphia: Lea & Febiger, 1985. With permission from Lippincott Williams & Wilkins, Philadelphia, PA.

Chapter 25

Fig. 25a: Koch, John C. "Laws of bone architecture." *American Journal of Anatomy*, 21: 177, © 1917, Wiley. Reprinted by permission of Wiley-Liss, Inc., a subsidiary of Wiley & Sons Inc.

Figs. 25b-25m: Havera, James Ronald. *Stress Line Analysis of the Base of the Skull in Animals and Man by the Split-Line Technique.* Master's Thesis; Chicago: 1961.

Chapter 29

Fig. 29a: Collection of Dr. Allan G. Brodie.

Fig. 29b: Collection of Dr. Allan G. Brodie.

Appendix II:

Endnotes

Chapters 3 and 13
The section "Reflex Control of the Airway," Chapter 3, "Functional Evolution of the Larynx," and the section "Growth Behavior of the Hyoid Bone," Chapter 13, "Muscle Physiology of Head and Neck Region: Internal," are essentially the same, as Dr. Allan G. Brodie used the information in both lectures. Fig. 3h and Fig. 13b are identical.

Chapter 8
In his paper *On the Growth of the Human Head from Birth to the Third Month,* Brodie writes, "In the mandible [of the newborn] the teeth were found to descend in their alignment from front to back with the central incisor closest to and second deciduous molar farthest from their positions of eruption. The first permanent molar crypt in this jaw, however, lay above the level of the deciduous teeth at the inner angle of the mandibular body and ramus."

Appendix III: Biography

Dr. Allan Gibson Brodie was born Oct. 31, 1897, in New York City.

After earning his DDS from the University of Pennsylvania in 1919, he began practicing dentistry in Newark, NJ, the next year.

In 1923, he married Vera Elizabeth Smock. They had three children: Allan Jr., Donald, and Anna (Olson).

Dr. Brodie studied under Edward H. Angle, the "father of orthodontics," at the Angle School of Orthodontics in Pasadena, CA, in 1925 and 1926, was considered Dr. Angle's best student, and matriculated in the school's final graduating class. Dr. Brodie, in turn, often referred to the Angles as his foster parents.

He returned to practice in Newark, but in 1929 he was invited by Dean Frederick B. Noyes to come to the University of Illinois College of Dentistry to organize its Department of Orthodontics—the first graduate orthodontics department established in the United States.

The *Journal of the Charles H. Tweed International Foundation* called Dr. Noyes' hiring of Dr. Brodie the beginning of "the golden age of orthodontics," and considered the department under Dr. Brodie "the West Point of orthodontics." The *Journal* also noted that the establishment of the Department of Orthodontics at the University of Illinois College of Dentistry "marked the fulfillment of Dr. Angle's lifelong ambition—to provide a broader and more scientific foundation for the practitioners of his specialty."

Dr. Brodie ran the department until 1966, and was Dean of the College from 1944 to 1956, while also maintaining a private practice, noting he believed in "practicing what you preach."

Dr. Brodie received his MS in anatomy and histology from the University in 1934, and his PhD in anatomy in 1940.

An internationally renowned orthodontics teacher, writer, and researcher, at various times Dr. Brodie served as President of the Chicago Association of Orthodontics; the Chicago Section of the International Association of Dental Research, and later of the entire IADR; the International Society of Craniofacial Biology; the annual Midwest Seminar of Dental Medicine (which he co-founded); and the Sigma Xi-Chicago Professional Campus Chapter.

He was a member of the Board of Scientific Advisors of the National Institute of Dental Research and the Research Scholarship Board of the National Institutes of Health; a member of the American Association of Orthodontics (AAO), where he established the Prize Essay Award to promote research; a founder of the Edward H. Angle Society of Orthodontia; and co-founder and for 42 years served as Associate Editor of *The Angle Orthodontist.*

Dr. Brodie's honors included being named the first Angle Memorial Lecturer in 1940; laureate of the George Villain Prize in 1947; a Joske Memorial Orator in Australia in 1954; recipient of the Callahan Gold Medal of the Ohio State Dental Society in 1957; recipient of the Ketcham Award of the AAO in 1959; Grieve Memorial Lecturer for the Canadian Dental Association in 1962; and, at the request of the U.S. Department of State, a Fulbright Professor of Orthodontics at the University of Nijmegen in the Netherlands in 1966.

He and his family always vacationed during the month of August at their summer home in Bear Lake, MI, where he pursued his favorite sport of trout fishing.

At the time of his death on Jan. 2, 1976, Dr. Brodie was writing his own book on orthodontics. Twenty-eight years later, *The Dentofacial Complex* at last has been published.